COMMON SENSE
Health
AND
Healing
DR. RICHARD SCHULZE

20 SIMPLE, EASY AND POWERFUL STEPS TO CREATE A NEW HEALTHY LIFE

D1281992

NATURAL HEALING
PUBLICATIONS
The VOICE of Dr. Richard Schulze

NATURAL HEALING
PUBLICATIONS

Published by Natural Healing Publications
P.O. Box 3628, Santa Monica, California 90408
1-877-TEACH-ME (832-2463)

Library of Congress Catalog Card Number: PENDING
<u>Common Sense: Health and Healing</u>
ISBN: 0-9671569-3-4

WARNING!

TABLE OF CONTENTS

INTRODUCTION
FOREWORD FROM DR. RICHARD SCHULZE — 8
How To Spot Imposters — 10
Dr. Schulze's Credentials — 19
CLINICAL CHARTS AND AFFIRMATIONS — 37
The First 5 Minutes in Dr. Schulze's Clinic — 39
The Faulty Mathematics of Medicine — 44
The Difference Between Natural Healing
and Medical Intervention — 48
The Fundamental Categories That
Determine Your Level of Health — 50

CHAPTER 1 — PURE WATER — 54
Why Should I?...Facts...How To Do It

CHAPTER 2 — FRESH JUICE — 58
Why Should I?...Facts...How To Do It

CHAPTER 3 — VEGAN FOOD — 64
Why Should I?...Facts...How To Do It
The Vegetarian Food Program
The Health Building Program

CHAPTER 4 — LIVE FOOD — 78
Why Should I?...Facts...How To Do It

CHAPTER 5 — BOWEL CLEANSING — 88
Why Should I?...Facts...How To Do It
The Intestinal Detoxification Program

TABLE OF CONTENTS

CHAPTER 6 **CLEANSING AND DETOXIFICATION 102**
Why Should I?...Facts...How To Do It
The 5 Day Cleansing and
Detoxification Program

CHAPTER 7 **BREATHE DEEPER** **118**
Why Should I?...Facts...How To Do It

CHAPTER 8 **STRETCHING, WALKING, MOVING 124**
Why Should I?...Facts...How To Do It

CHAPTER 9 **WATER THERAPY** **134**
Why Should I?...Facts...How To Do It

CHAPTER 10 **NATURAL CLOTHING** **140**
Why Should I?...Facts...How To Do It

CHAPTER 11 **NATURAL CLEANING** **144**
Why Should I?...Facts...How To Do It

CHAPTER 12 **STOP TELEVISION** **148**
Why Should I?...Facts...How To Do It

CHAPTER 13 **TRASHING** **152**
Why Should I?...Facts...How To Do It

TABLE OF CONTENTS

CHAPTER 14 **RELAXATION** **158**
Why Should I?...Facts...How To Do It

CHAPTER 15 **EXPRESS YOURSELF** **166**
Why Should I?...Facts...How To Do It

CHAPTER 16 **HELP OTHERS** **170**
Why Should I?...Facts...How To Do It

CHAPTER 17 **LAUGH MORE** **172**
Why Should I?...Facts...How To Do It

CHAPTER 18 **MORE SEX** **174**
Why Should I?...Facts...How To Do It

CHAPTER 19 **LISTENING TO YOURSELF** **180**
Why Should I?...Facts...How To Do It

CHAPTER 20 **LOVE LIFE** **182**
Why Should I?...Facts...How To Do It

CHAPTER 21 **FINAL THOUGHTS** **196**
Final Hour Regrets
Poem from Dr. Schulze's Dead Patients

> **"Healing Disease and Getting Well is very simple and easy.**
> *All you have to do is...*
> **STOP what you did that made you sick in the first place...and START new habits that will heal you and create vibrant health.**
> *And the miracle happens..."*

This book is Dedicated to

Adam Loef, my friend, for your great support of my work, your great leadership in running the American Botanical Pharmacy, and your great focus and clarity, which has helped get my message to millions, and especially for your willingness to learn more and grow more every day.

Anisha Jones for your great love, personal support, courage, passion, and for keeping my spirit and integrity alive.

Arthur, my son, who keeps me young and is the future of healthy and loving children.

To my graphics team, Adam again, Ty, Gregg, Paul, and Josh. Without your big effort and some sleepless nights, this book would not have been printed.

To Dr. Rocannon MacGregor, my longtime friend and accomplice in many natural healing adventures. We have traveled many roads together that most people wouldn't go down. What fun!

To Devamarga, Peter Jackson-Main, and all of my practicing students and health crusaders all over the world, I send my love and support. Keep up the great work.

To Hilda, Thea, Leonel, Marlene, Chad and Louis, Thanks.

To Jack for your assistance with my crusade and to Buddy for your friendship.

And finally to Dr. Bruce Parker for keeping my back feeling great while sitting on my butt for a month writing this book.

Dr. Richard Schulze

FOREWORD
TO THE FIRST EDITION
BY DR. RICHARD SCHULZE AUGUST 2002

From Webster's College Dictionary, latest edition:
Bullshit (bool' shit) [Slang] noun. *Foolish, exaggerated, or boastful talk;* **_NONSENSE_** –bull **shit-ting – to talk nonsense**
(Somewhat vulgar)

Almost every single day of my adult life I meet people that say to me, "you should read this <u>health</u> book," or, "I saw an <u>herb</u> book that you would really like," or, *God forbid*, "I'd like you to read my new <u>nutrition</u> book." My usual response to this person is that I won't like it. In fact I'd say that chances are about 99% that I will hate it. The simple reason I won't like it is because it is bullshit. Sure, I could have said *fiction,* which means something *made up* or *imagined*, but that sounds too clean. In my three decades of practice I have seen people die clutching these healing fairy tale books on their death beds, still believing, still hoping right up to the end, turning blue gasping for their last breath, writhing in pain, suffocating in their vomit, and eventually dying, so I prefer to say bullshit, because these books stink and their authors are full of shit!

If I want fiction I will read the Adventures of Huckleberry Finn or Moby Dick. At least I am pre-warned that this is fiction, make believe, a fun story, entertainment.

A classic example of fiction being passed off as truth is the business section of any book store. They have shelves and tables piled high with books entitled "Get Rich Quick" or "How to Become a Millionaire". The only laugh is that about 99% of the authors aren't rich or millionaires themselves. Don't you think that if they really knew how to make a million bucks that they would have done it first themselves? So after you remove J. Paul Getty and a handful of other actual millionaire authors from this group, you end up with tens of thousands of books that people purchase to learn how to get rich, but the author hasn't a clue either. Think about it: if the author actually knew how to make millions, and did make millions, why would they be wasting time writing books and not be busy making millions? They sure as heck wouldn't be writing books telling you how to be their competitor.

Have you ever seen the bumper sticker or heard the wonderful simple statement QUESTION AUTHORITY Question Authority literally means to question the author's *power*.

<u>My Point:</u> I am referring to the thousands and thousands of health, natural healing and herbal medicine books available in book stores and health food stores all over America, in fact all over the world. The reason I don't like 99% of these books is because they are *fiction* being passed off as *truth,* and people die because of this.

FIVE TIPS
ON SPOTTING A BOOK ON HEALTH AND HEALING THAT WON'T GET YOU WELL!

Or... How to *judge* a book by its cover ... or more accurately, by it's *author*.

The first place to look when checking out any health book is the inside flaps of the cover or the back outside cover. This is where you will usually find the few paragraphs about the author. Publishers often hide or quickly gloss over the author's credentials. This is usually because they have none, or at least none that are <u>specifically</u> relevant to the book's subject. The following is a checklist I have given to many students and patients over the years to help them evaluate the healing potential of any health book.

HOW TO SPOT IMPOSTERS | TIP NUMBER ONE

The Author should have extensive **PERSONAL EXPERIENCE** with their own program, using it on themselves.

I would actually prefer that the author has been sick, really sick, if not dying, and then developed their program to save their own ass. I know that for me personally, my passion, enthusiasm, intensity and drive all stems from the fact that medical doctors told me I would be dead before I was twenty and that I desperately went on to figure out how to heal myself from what the medical doctors called an incurable disease. FEAR is an incredibly potent motivational tool. OK, so everyone is not as lucky as me to have been born sick and then have the illumination and education of healing themselves but damn it, I want some serious dues being paid by the author, at least a close relative dying or a pet dog suffering.

And I don't want to hear about any health or healing program that the author hasn't completely immersed themselves in either, and for years. I am so sick of listening to *virgin sex counselors.* If my life is on the line I want some damn personal experience. I don't think that is too much to ask.

A Computer Software Analogy

There is nothing worse than upgrading to the latest release of your favorite software only to discover that it doesn't work very well, won't interface with most of your other programs and ends up corrupting and destroying data files and crashing your computer. **This only happens because the author or manufacturer didn't test their work long enough.** This is why most computer users today are skeptical of *hot new software releases, upgrades and operating systems* and want to see the programs field-tested for a year or so before they load it onto their computer and waste their hard-earned money and their time and risk ruining their computer's *health.* See my point and the similarity?

So I want, I demand, that these health and healing authors have done their own program a 100 times over, working out all of the kinks and glitches, and I want them to have done it 100 times more intensely than they are suggesting that I should do it in their book, and I want them to have done it in a hundred different ways, with a hundred different variables. I want them to have GONE TOO FAR with their program, to have hurt themselves and made themselves sick, to have puked and pooped their pants and to have learned what is too much and, more importantly, what is too little and what won't work. I want them to personally know their program inside and out, have done it on their relatives, their friends or their cat, until they really know deep down in their bone marrow, their soul, what they are talking about. If they haven't, you guessed it, it's bullshit.

How To Spot Imposters TIP NUMBER TWO

The Author should have had some kind of **SPECIFIC TRAINING** that is specific to their programs in the book.

If not then I would at least like some explanation of how they received this message of healing knowledge. I fully accept having a revelation or spending a year alone in the woods. It doesn't have to be a formal education of any kind, but I would like some relevant personal background as to why they feel they are qualified to write a book on this subject before I literally put my ass on the enema line. (By the way, I do not accept AA, BA or MA degrees, or even a doctorate in any non-related study.) How many books do you see in which the author has to list their non-related degrees like they should get some special appreciation or credibility from the reader that their parents sent them to college instead of getting a job. What does their masters degree in fine arts have to do with my gall bladder?

Also, don't get fooled by other authors that have great credentials and training in a very similar-sounding field or incredible education and degrees but in a <u>closely-related</u> field. This is very common in herbal medicine and natural healing. For instance, although botany is the science of all plants and then categorizing them by variations in their flowers, and pharmacology and pharmacognosy are the study of the chemicals in plants and how they affect your metabolism, and ethnobotany is considered the study of how our ancestors used herbs, a professor in any of these related fields usually has many *opinions, theories* and *hypotheses* that they discovered in the *library* or on the *internet* about how plants are used for healing. But none of their herbal theories will stand a chance in hell of dissolving a stone out of your gall bladder or kidney using herbs.

I personally know the authors of hundreds of published books on natural healing and herbal medicine. I have hired many of them to teach at colleges I advise all over the world. They are experts in their particular field, but then they go and write a book on herbal first aid when their expertise is actually plant identification.

In the same vein I know of a popular book written by an herbalist that specialized in making herbal cosmetics, hand lotions and hair conditioners, but they needed money so they wrote a book on healing cancer and other degenerative diseases with herbs. These are the most dangerous authors of all so read about their credentials very carefully. Your life might just depend on it.

And if it happens to be a Medical Doctor that is writing the book on natural healing or herbal medicine, then this is even more points off. This is as ludicrous as a career criminal writing a book on honesty and morality. Unless this MD has had some amazing lightning strike enlightenment as to how they were exploded off the path of medical mayhem, and then they fully admit that they now know that the majority of all medical doctors are greedy, unthinking butchers, and that the practice of modern medicine and hospitals are responsible for killing far more people than they help, and that they apologize for any wrong deeds they did during their unconscious past, unless they prostrate themselves . . . . . . their work has no credibility and they should write a book on surgery, chemotherapy, or antibiotics.

I am dead serious on this issue: natural healing books written by medical doctors who have studied only disease and have no education in health, nutrition, natural healing and herbology, are, you guessed it, bullshit!

HOW TO SPOT IMPOSTERS — TIP NUMBER THREE

The Author should have <u>CLINICAL EXPERIENCE</u> successfully helping hundreds, if not thousands, of people heal themselves and get well using their program.

Unlike most people, I don't give a damn if the book is a New York Times bestseller and sold over a million copies. Pet rocks made millions of dollars too. No one ever said that the average consumer was a good judge of a quality product. People love fads and healing fads often run out of gas very quickly for the simple reason that they do not work.

What I want to know is that the author instructed numerous people on how to follow the program and that these people healed their diseases, healed their illnesses, healed themselves and then built powerful health and remained disease free, <u>longer than the average person treated medically</u>.

This is where the vast majority of health authors fall short and fail this test. Even if they have healed themselves of a major disease using their program, and even if medical doctors said what they had was incurable, it could be a fluke. Some people win the lottery but the odds are ten million to one that you won't. People heal themselves of cancer drinking beer and eating hot dogs and cotton candy, but it's extremely rare. So I want to see their personal experience about their personal healing miracle and the program that they then developed put into practice, to see if it works on anyone else besides themselves. Is this program really the better, more effective and literally miraculous new improved Bowel Detoxification Program, or is it just gas?

During any doctor's education their brain gets filled with millions of ideas and so-called facts, hypotheses and supposed proven theories, and also some good valid programs, but to the student they all look exactly the same. It is impossible for the student to differentiate between fact and fiction. <u>This is where clinical experience comes to the rescue</u>. Helping real people, with real diseases, get real well, helps uncover and weed out all the ineffective programs really fast. This is when patients educate the student into a doctor.

One of America's greatest natural healers, the late Dr. John R. Christopher, a Mormon doctor from Utah whom I apprenticed with, was a rare example of a great doctor. Rare because he actually helped thousands and thousands of people all across America heal their diseases, even the so-called *incurable* ones. Dr. Christopher was well aware who his teachers were and often would say that "5% of what I know I learned in school, and 95% of what I know I learned from my patients in the clinic." This very wise man and great herbal doctor knew where real knowledge comes from.

There are many incredible scientists, botanists, pharmacologists, herbalists, master herbalists and medical herbalists out there with many degrees. They teach at medical universities all over the world and lecture everywhere. They can almost always be found speaking at the big important health conferences, expositions and hip natural gatherings. They write numerous magazine articles, design formulas for big name herbal and nutrition companies and often are founding members of natural, herbal and health organizations. They have spent countless hours hob knobbing with the other gurus of health. But their work is all hearsay, third-hand gossip, because they have no practical, clinical experience. They simply never had any patients.

So here is what I want. I want to see their healing results, they have *hopefully* personally experienced and claim to be valid in their book, repeated often. I want a minimum number of people, over a minimum period of time. I say the minimum should be 5 years of clinical practice and 4,000 patient visits. This is simply because that in a clinical setting with real live sick people knocking at your door, you are quickly forced to separate what works from what doesn't; after all it's a matter of life and death. Also, by this point most good doctors have thrown out the majority of their books, dropped most of what they learned in school, thrown out their stethoscopes and sphygmomanometers and softened their "I know it all" egos and have been humbled by their patients who didn't respond and died. More importantly they have learned "what works" from their patients who are still alive. Now they truly *know* what works, and what is (you guessed it again) bullshit.

An Insightful Analogy

What if you got on an airplane with only one pilot, and before takeoff this pilot announced that they have many degrees in aeronautics, have been to flight training school, spent endless hours on the computer flight simulator, but have actually never been aboard an airplane before and never actually flown one before. I hope you would see all of the passengers running and screaming and diving out of the exit doors. Health and Healing books written by authors with no clinical experience are no different.

HOW TO SPOT IMPOSTERS TIP NUMBER FOUR

The Program should be <u>SIMPLE</u> and should make <u>COMMON SENSE</u>. It should not heal one organ while making another organ sick. No tradeoffs.

All healing programs should be simple. If it is too complicated, then the author needs more time in the clinic, just like a fine young port needs more time to age in the bottle. The programs are simply not refined enough yet. Check back with them in 5 or 10 more years and see if they have got it down yet. I find that the complicated programs are written by people who are not focusing on the fundamentals of health and healing, but are instead written and designed by people who are still focusing on killing, or curing, *disease.* Unfortunately many authors, <u>especially ones who went to medical school</u>, are often so ruined by their *education* that they will never be able to see things from a simple and natural perspective. They will never be able to be natural healers because they are so focused on killing your disease, they will miss the simple cause of it that is right in front of their nose.

The program should make common sense, too. Most people's programs don't. If it doesn't feel right to you, that is because it isn't right. All great healing programs make common sense.

Lastly, the health program should not heal one organ while making another organ sick. No tradeoffs. How many times have you heard that the medical doctors got all the cancer, cut it all out with surgery, burnt it all out with radiation and poisoned all the malignant cells to death with chemotherapy, but the patient died. Let's see, get cut, get burned, get poisoned, pay one hundred thousand dollars, and die. Call me silly, but this doesn't seem like a very good program. Modern medicine is also full of drug tradeoffs like take this pill and you'll be able to eat and digest anything, but . . . you might get liver cancer. Or take this medicine to help your liver, but . . . it might kill Kidney cells. Or you begin to take a beta blocker drug for your irregular heartbeat, but if you forget to take your pills once you start on the drug, you will die from a massive heart attack.

Medicine is full of dangerous tradeoffs, but so are many natural healing programs. Many *natural* doctors suggest making Liver and Gall Bladder flushes with Cola soda pop, but last I checked Cola isn't what I consider natural. Other *natural* doctors suggest flushing out your bowel with powerful salt-laden flushes, but if you have high blood pressure, this flush could kill you. ALL healing programs should also be nutritious and healthy. I know that sounds almost too simple to understand, so I will repeat it:

All *healing programs* should be *healthy*.

How To Spot Imposters TIP NUMBER FIVE

Beware of DEAD AUTHORS

Being dead doesn't necessarily invalidate the author's work, but in many cases the work has been altered, weakened, made more politically correct or even legally safe to protect their surviving family and heirs. After all, the author was probably a clinically hardened radical natural healer and is now almost considered a politically incorrect dinosaur. Unfortunately, the author is no longer around to protect their work from this type of corruption, so all they can do is spin in their grave while people get sicker using their weakened programs and *updated* herbal formulae. Meanwhile their surviving relatives cash in their royalty checks.

Many of the most popular books on natural healing and herbal medicine sold today were written by people who are now dead. Often the book was actually written or *updated* (watered down) by the daughter, or son, or niece, nephew, or some relative. Don't laugh. This is the case with many of the most popular books out there. Many of these books are also compiled by ghostwriters who take the person's notes after they are dead and literally make a book out of it. I even know of one that was compiled by the next door neighbor who had no experience in the field at all but was good on the computer.

Watch out for books that have been updated with flashy new covers. I have found that most of these are politically correct, watered-down versions of the doctor's original work, with all the effective, but possibly *illegal* or *legally compromising* healing programs, forced out of the book by the publisher's legal staff or some gutless and wimpy relatives. I have also often seen great doctors' effective herbal formulas have ingredients *removed* and natural healing programs *modernized* because supposedly *times have changed.* Well, maybe times have changed, but the human body hasn't.

If you believe in an author, but they are dead, either try to find old copies of their books that were published while they were alive or find their top students, apprentices and interns and see what they are up to.

Why do I care if you buy a useless book? Why is this a problem?

Probably because I spent too many years in the clinic and I have a soft spot for dying patients who are desperately trying to stay alive following bullshit programs. Call me a bleeding heart but I dislike anyone who preys on the sick and takes their nest egg in the final days of their life. Of course medical doctors are the most famous for this behavior.

If I haven't been obvious enough so far I will clarify it even further. The best case scenario is that you are just wasting your hard-earned money and what little spare time you have buying and reading these worthless books. Worse yet, you could make yourself very ill (as I have done many times) by following *theoretical* programs. You could be the first person to actually take this author seriously and follow their program. If you want to be an astronaut or explorer, fine, but if you want to get well, you could get sick instead. Luckily most of these experimental programs just caused me projectile vomiting, lightheadedness and really becoming an astronaut for a few days, learning first-hand the laws of rectal jet propulsion.

But the worst case scenario is that you are very ill, have little time left and the medical doctors have taken all of your money and told you to go home and die. You are hoping that the book you are reading will help you make your final turnaround. Instead you get worse and die.

DR. SCHULZE'S CREDENTIALS AND QUALIFICATIONS TO WRITE THIS BOOK

Now you are aware that most books on health, natural healing and herbal medicine aren't worth the paper they are written on. You also have some tips to deduce the credibility of authors, and therefore the possible effectiveness and safety of their suggested programs.

At this point I think it is only fair that I put myself through the same exact acid test. Therefore the following is a detailed explanation of my credentials and qualifications, scrutinized by the same standards I suggested for other authors.

MY PERSONAL HEALING EXPERIENCE
WITH NATURAL HEALING AND HERBAL MEDICINE

Having healed myself of a life-threatening disease and numerous supposedly *incurable* injuries, the following is an account of my extensive personal *first*-hand knowledge of natural self healing.

MY DEATH SENTENCE

My father died in my arms when I was only 11 years old. He was only 55. He had a massive heart attack, but he died very slowly. It was torturous for him physically, and for me emotionally, because it took him about three hours to die. He was in severe pain, he sweated so profusely he soaked the sheet of the bed into almost a puddle, he vomited, lost bladder and bowel control, cried, screamed at some points, and all of a sudden he went quiet, all the pain stopped, and he was peaceful. He looked into my eyes and said, "I'm Dead," and then slumped into my arms for the last time. I could see his tremendous fear, not so much of dying but more of what was going to happen to me.

My mother was not prepared for this in any way. She went downhill from this day on and died herself of a massive heart attack only a few years later, also at the age of 55. I was then only 14.

I lived on the streets, in communes and in the slums of big cities. I ate out of many a garbage can and, by the age of sixteen, I was having severe pain in my left arm, left jaw and in my heart. I would pass out at least once a day and up to 4 times a day after having massive heart palpitations. Eventually I went to the hospital, where they ran many tests and ultimately diagnosed me with a deformed heart and deformed heart valves. They said that without starting on cardiac drugs immediately and having open-heart corrective surgery, I would be dead in only a few years. They said I would be dead by 20 because my weak, deformed heart and valves would not be able to pump sufficient blood to an adult body.

I asked my doctor if there was anything else I could possibly do, besides cutting my ribs in half and cutting into my heart. The thought of this horrible, gruesome surgery scared me to death. I asked him, what if I exercised like mad, what if I ate differently (because health food stores were starting to pop up around town), what if I prayed . . . ? He looked at me and said, "I'm sorry, this is a physical deformity and only surgery will keep you from dying".

I was scared to death, scared of death, and checked myself into the hospital. I met another teenager in the hospital and we became friends. He had almost the exact same problem as I did and was scheduled to have the same surgery as me about two weeks before mine. I will always remember when my doctor, who was also his doctor, came into my room and told me that my friend had died on the table. I was stunned, shocked, filled with rage, hate and anger. I got dressed and ran out of that hospital that day, and I never looked back.

I knew that I was dying, but I also knew that if I stayed in the hospital, the same doctor that killed my friend was going to kill me in two weeks time. It was like the French foreign legion when they say, *march or die,* so I marched. Running out of the hospital, literally running for my life, was the beginning of my journey, my adventure into self-healing, into natural healing.

THE NEXT THREE YEARS

I immediately started talking to anyone and everyone, telling them that I was dying and asking them if they had any natural suggestions that could help me. Everyone I met did indeed have some sort of suggestion, so I compiled a journal of them because there were so many, **AND I DID THEM ALL!**

FOOD

I grew up in a German household where we ate blood for breakfast, lunch, dinner and dessert. I rarely saw a vegetable and if one mistakenly did end up on my plate, well, I would scoop it off and give it to my dog, who wouldn't eat it either. OK, potatoes, we ate potatoes. By 16 my cholesterol level was well over 300. Right around this time most medical doctors agreed that coronary artery disease was a disease of the elderly. But this was also the early years of the Vietnam War and 18 and 19 year-olds were getting bullet and shrapnel wounds to the chest. The war surgeons were finding advanced coronary artery disease in the chests of teenagers, so the medical world was seeing something shocking. They were just starting to think about changing their minds about coronary artery disease. This previously almost exclusive disease of the elderly was now being seen in teenagers. This was due to a new era in America, the fast food hamburger chains that literally didn't exist a decade earlier.

Anyway, a friend suggested that I stop eating red meat. I did, and I felt better. Shortly thereafter I stopped eating chicken and fish and became what I refer to as a lacto, lacto, lacto, lacto, ovo, ovo, ovo, ovo, ovo, vegetarian because I lived on vanilla milk shakes, chocolate milk, eggs, cheese omelettes, toasted cheese sandwiches, and ice cream. I felt a lot better, my heart palpitations were reduced by half in both number and severity, but I was obviously still having a cholesterol problem.

So the next step to try and reduce my blood fat and cholesterol level even further was to stop eating all foods that contained cholesterol. In other words, to stop eating dairy products and eggs. I remember that day well. I thought I was going to die of starvation, because when I finished cleaning all the dairy products and eggs out of my refrigerator, **THERE WAS NOTHING LEFT IN IT!** I ended up starving for a few weeks because I still wasn't going to eat any stinkin' vegetables.

In a few weeks I started getting the hang of it and in a few months I was in hog heaven, eating like a vegan pig. That was over 30 years ago and I have been a vegan vegetarian ever since. Over the next few years I discovered juicing, sprouting, and fermenting. I went exclusively on raw foods for about a year and a half and I also discovered grain burgers, baked potatoes, pasta and hundreds of other dishes of substance.

The bottom line is that I have personally made the transition from my parents' food program that was killing me to a new healthy food program that healed my disease. I was then able to thrive on this food program and maintain it for over 30 years, staying disease free and in great health. And enjoying every meal.

COLON CLEANSING

During the first few months of my new healing program, I heard much talk in the health circles about colon cleansing. I had ignored all of this bowel talk as long as I could but eventually realized that I could not be healthy, and have a healthy heart, while I was constipated. I had noticed, as my food program was changing, that I was having more bowel movements, but I had been constipated since I was a kid and I was an excellent candidate for some deep colon cleaning. Heck, I would have settled for a guaranteed one bowel movement a day.

I remember as a kid, once a week on Sunday my Dad would go into the bathroom with the Sunday newspaper. He would spend an hour or more in there squeezing and grunting and would eventually come out and the smell of death would permeate the house. I would go in shortly after him and try to have my once-a-week bowel movement too. Sometimes no matter how much I pushed and squeezed, nothing would come out. Look, I come from a long line of constipated Germans. So if and when I did have a bowel movement, and that wasn't every Sunday, it would be these hard, black, granite balls that would explode out of my rear end, sink fast in the toilet, and they were so hard I used to think they might chip the china toilet. I remember my brother could go a month without a bowel movement. I remember once or twice a year as a kid my mom would have to take him to the hospital and the doctors would have to put on rubber gloves and go into my brother's rectum with their fingers and pull old hard dried fecal matter, (He will kill me if he reads this book!) Bottom line (pun intended): we were a very constipated family.

So when I set out to clean my colon I did it like I did everything else on my health program, with intensity, passion, gusto and more intensity. I gave myself over 100 enemas, of all different kinds and variations. I used every natural and herbal bowel tonic of the era but I can say that most of them were no good. When I found one that would work, I often would take 100 capsules, the entire bottle. I remember creating my own program of 100 capsules of herbal bowel tonic, two quarts of fresh squeezed apple juice and 1 quart of home made prune juice, ALL BEFORE NOON. That day I was way up on an extension ladder painting when the boss asked me if I could reach the top of the peak of the house. I reached up, stretched a little and crapped my pants. I took my pants off in the car and then my bowels moved again right in the seat of my car. I ran in the house with only a towel wrapped around me and had my first deep experience of bowel cleansing. I was a pioneer, a cosmonaut. I was paying my dues.

The bottom line is that after 15 good years of bowel cleansing, many enemas, some high colonics, herbal implants and inventing my own herbal bowel formulae and using them consistently for 12 years, my colon has worked perfectly ever since. I now have 2 to 3 bowel movements a day, reflecting the 2 to 3 meals that I eat a day.

CLEANSING AND DETOXIFICATION

Besides colon cleansing I also learned that everyone should do routine cleansing and detoxification programs. And if you're ill, and I was seriously ill, then a person should do their cleansing and detoxification programs for a longer duration and with more intensity.

I started out with water fasting and found it uncomfortable and unnecessary. I also found it difficult because I worked out physically quite a lot because that was part of my healing program too. Maybe if someone is just fasting and lying around then water fasting is alright, but when you are active and doing a lot of other cleansing and purifying routines I felt it not sensible when done for more than 2 - 3 days. I then upgraded to juice fasting, which I could do for longer periods of time, achieving the same detoxifying results, and getting the nutritional support I needed. Most importantly, I could follow my other natural healing regiments and routines at the same time.

I personally did two 30-day juice fasts and one 60-day juice fast. I have also done over 50 week-long juice fasts. From this experience I developed my 5 Day Cleansing and Detoxification Program. During these various cleansing and detoxification programs I also investigated and experienced using numerous herbal formulae to enhance the cleansing process. I also investigated Hydrotherapy and have visited hydrotherapy clinics, trained at some and completed their programs all over the world.

I have formed groups where we investigated liver flushing, gallbladder flushing, kidney and bladder flushing, lung purging and skin detoxification.

The bottom line is that I have personally experienced numerous cleansing and detoxification programs and flushes and have done many of them to extreme and intense levels.

MOVEMENT

Having a deformed heart I quickly learned that exercise was going to have to now be a part of my life, forever. But I am easily bored so I needed to find some type of exercise that would also keep me entertained. Martial Arts appealed to me and I have been involved in the practice of it since I was a teenager, and then later in life taught it for years. I also found that hatha yoga helped my healing dramatically, and I trained extensively in that too. I have trained with professional trainers and have worked my entire life to make moving fun, or else I quit.

The bottom line is that I have been involved in numerous types of aerobic and anaerobic exercise, stretching and flexibility since I was a kid.

EMOTIONAL AND SPIRITUAL

Obviously I had to do a tremendous amount of emotional and spiritual healing. Even though it would seem that my parents simply died when I was a young child, to me, dead or not, it was pure abandonment.

Then, growing up on the streets, at least to start, well, I had a lot of issues. To add to the list I also had plenty of *"why me?"* issues because after all, I WAS DYING.

I took a course in Psychology 101 and dabbled in psychotherapy sessions, but all of it seemed so tame compared to my very aggressive and intensive natural healing program. Oh, it had value, but I didn't want to spend my whole life in psychotherapy, I wanted to be well NOW!

So the treatment plan I followed was much more of a new age psychotherapy treatment program which included Geshtalt, Reichien, Rebirthing, Neuro-Linguistic Programming, Reverend Ike, Positive Affirmations – all of it explosive, cathartic kind of work. I had a truckload of existential nausea and I needed to get right, and I did.

I went on to train in most of these mentioned arts and used them extensively with my patients.

I also followed a spiritual path that is unorthodox and unorganized, unlike most religions, which I still practice and follow today.

Most importantly I discovered that anger and hate were killing me and that I had to learn to be loving if I wanted to heal my heart. You can't have a healthy heart, or any health for that matter, unless you first love yourself, and secondly your life. And then, of course, others.

The bottom line: I am no longer the physically and emotionally constipated German, pissed-off, angry kid I once was. To create my metamorphosis to the person I am today, it took a lot of emotional and spiritual healing, and a lot of self-acceptance and love.

THREE YEARS LATER

After about three years on all of these programs I was about 19. Remember, the doctors said I would be dead by 20. So I made an appointment to see the same medical doctor that gave me that death sentence. Was he shocked to see me! I was the picture of health. He first wondered where I had disappeared to three years ago and what happened to me. He asked me how I was feeling, and I said great, but he still suggested the surgery. I asked him if he would re-run all the tests and see if I had changed, if my disease had changed, if my heart had changed. He said it wouldn't have because it was a physical deformity and that couldn't change. But he said he would like some new tests, x-rays and cardiogram anyway to update the further degeneration of my disease, so I spent the next few days in and out of the hospital.

A few days later I was asked to come in for a consultation with him and when I walked into the room he had an absolutely shocked look on his face. He said the new test results showed no heart disease at all and that if he hadn't had my previous x-rays from three years earlier he wouldn't have believed it with his own eyes. I asked why and he said because **your heart and your heart valves are NOT deformed anymore, they are NORMAL**! I asked him if he was interested in what I had done that healed my heart and started to mention my health programs and he just rolled his eyes. He immediately interrupted me and said "I don't know how your heart undeformed itself but if there is one thing that I do know it is that it had NOTHING to do with your health program." He was in disbelief and in denial and the tests and pictures didn't lie. It was more than he could bear. I felt that he would have much rather I had died. My healing was shaking his belief system. His shaky medical house of cards was crumbling down, and I could tell that he wanted me out of his office and out of his sight. Little did I know then that three decades later this same attitude of medical denial and fear of healing miracles would have me arrested.

So here, three years later, after three years on my healing adventure, I had actually healed my heart and my heart disease. I knew at that moment that your body could heal itself of anything, if you just gave it a chance to do so. And the best way to give it this chance was to create a healthy lifestyle.

MY SUPPOSEDLY *INCURABLE* INJURIES

HAND AND KNEE

The following is transcribed from a live Dr. Schulze speaking engagement at the Church of the Living Word, North Hills, California April 22, 2000.

When I was in the clinic years later, there was a lot of healings and miracles around me and an occasional explosion too. One day there was an explosion and fire in the lab and boiling, flaming oil poured all over my right hand. It burnt my hand almost off, it curled up into a ball, but I was a tough young cocky natural healer and I thought, No Problem. I thought I could heal this in a few days, but after a few days I realized I had done some serious damage to my hand.

A friend of mine who was an MD told me he knew a man, another MD who was a burn specialist, especially with hands, and that he was interested in natural healing and that he would give me his opinion. So I went to see this doctor and he looked at my hand and he said, this is a very serious burn. You have a fourth degree burn, he said, and I hadn't heard of 4th degree. I'd heard of 1st, 2nd and 3rd, but not 4th. I said what's 4th, and he said that is when all the tissue is dead down to the bone. He said I had even cooked some of the bone. I said that it didn't feel that bad, and he said that's because you have burnt all the nerves, that they were dead too. And I said that it still didn't feel that bad and he took an implement and pulled all the flesh off one of my fingers like a cooked chicken and opened up a hole right to my middle finger bone. I don't want to hold this finger up all by itself…Not in Church…and he opened up a hole right to the bone. All the little tendons and all the little ligaments were cooked and burnt and even the bone was charred.

I could feel myself feeling a little faint, and then he took a clamp and he put it on my thumb where he very easily slid the casing of my thumb off. It was cooked and that put me into a state of shock that I will never forget. And he said, you don't understand, you need a skin graft, your skin is gone, buddy. He said, you need to sew skin onto your hand. And I thought, I believe that, because it's gone now, it was for sure gone now, and I said OK, I'll take a skin graft.

The next thing I remember is that the doctor said "will you take down your pants" and I thought, I know I am in Hollywood, but this sounds weird. And so I thought OK, I took down my pants and he had a magic marker and he was drawing something on my butt, and I thought this is a bit weird and I said, what are you doing, and he said this is where we're going to take the skin to sew on your hand.

Immediately I remember having that exact same feeling that I had in the hospital when my friend died and I pulled my pants up really quick and ran out of the hospital. This doctor almost had me believing again that my body wouldn't heal itself, AND THEN MY NATURAL HEALING ALARM WENT OFF IN MY HEAD. Hey, it's bad enough to have a burned-off hand but now he's going to cut the skin off my beautiful rear-end, and I thought, I know my body can heal itself. I tried to tell him about my heart, but he didn't want to listen . . . . . So I left, and in thirty days I had skin covering this hand and it was starting to work again, and I went back and showed him and he had that same look on his face that my first heart doctor did. I could actually see him jolt in his chair, and he said, what have you done? And I said I think my hand grew back, I think I grew skin back and he said the same thing, that it was a miracle. I said I know, would you want to hear what I did, and he said yes. . . . . .and so I began to tell him about the 147 things that I did...the running outside even though it was bleeding through my sling, drinking carrot juice and then soaking my hand in the carrot pulp, drinking wheat grass juice, soaking my hand in the wheat grass juice, all the herbs I used, the prayer, the meditation, the long story, the whole program, and I could see that same look in his face.

And I almost thought he was writing, "delusional, mildly schizophrenic" in his chart when he said, "You don't understand, I have been doing this work, doing surgical skin grafting onto severe burns for thirty-five years. I have never, ever, ever, ever, once, seen someone grow back their skin, especially when all the skin was dead, FOURTH DEGREE BURNS!" Because you can't grow skin from thin air, you can't grow skin from osteoblasts, or bone cells. You have to have skin there to grow skin, and he said, "This is impossible, but somehow you have managed it." Then he said, "I don't understand it and how is this possible?"

I looked him straight in the eyes and said, you have spent your whole life, your entire career, sewing people's rear-ends onto their hand. And you are very good at doing that, but there are *other ways to heal your body*, there is a healing beyond sewing rear-ends to hands. There is a healing that your body can do if you're willing to take responsibility and create a healing lifestyle, which is what I did, and I have a brand new hand with skin all over it and it works great, without a skin graft. I walked out and I can still see this medical doctor sitting there, stunned, shocked, perplexed, mystified.

Doctors know very little about the ability of the human body to repair itself, mainly because they have spent the last 100 years getting in the way of this natural healing process.

A few years later I decided to be a skier. And I was really enjoying it because it was quiet and I would go down these hills and then I started entering some of the races and my ego got involved, and then I started doing the NASTAR Amateur races and I remember I was at Deer Valley, Utah, going around my last bamboo, I was tucked all the way down and I heard this big "POP"! I remember going face-first into the snow, and that was all I remember.

Later I heard from witnesses and the members of the ski patrol that I turned into an incredible human snowball. I woke up in the hospital where the Doctor was holding my leg in his hand by cupping it under my knee. It was just dangling, and I could feel nothing there. He said, you have pretty much destroyed your knee. He said, I need to get you on a plane, in a splint, back to Los Angeles as fast as you can where you can go to the best orthopedic surgeons and have your knee put back together. And I said, fine.

I flew back to Los Angeles and went to the biggest and most famous orthopedic surgery group here in L.A., the one that does all the sports stars from around the world. We all know who they are. And they told me, you have really destroyed your knee. You have torn out and broken all of your medial collateral ligaments on the inside of your knee. You have blown out all the interior cruciate ligaments in the middle of your knee, you've torn your cartilage, you've torn your meniscus, you need surgery. And I had that feeling again. I said well, Doc, let me tell you about my heart and <u>now my hand,</u> and he listened a little bit, but he said, you don't understand. He said, I deal with professional athletes, football players, baseball players, basketball players, hockey players, tennis players.. and when I see these kinds of injuries, if you don't have surgery, **YOU WILL NEVER, EVER WALK AGAIN!**

Not a very positive man. I said, but I think my body knows how to heal itself. And he said, are you telling me that a ligament that's down here and one that's up there, 6 inches apart, will know how to find each other, grow together and reconnect themselves? And I thought, well, my heart knew what to do, and my hand knew what to do, why wouldn't my knee? And he, again, convinced me that this was such a severe injury that I needed to have surgery and I said OK. And he said that in fact it's so bad we're going to have to take ligaments out of a dead body, a cadaver, and sew them into your leg. And I remember MY NATURAL HEALING ALARM WENT OFF AGAIN. HERE IS ANOTHER MEDICAL DOCTOR, A VERY SMART MEDICAL DOCTOR, TELLING ME THAT MY BODY ISN'T CAPABLE OF HEALING ITSELF!

"I'm not going to do this!" I yelled. And his final words to me were, **"YOU WILL NEVER WALK AGAIN"**. And I thought, I'll be walking within a couple weeks. Well, in a month I couldn't walk AT ALL, I was totally crippled. In two months I had a severe limp, and I could barely drag the leg and not put much weight on it, but I started doing all my routines to it, going to the gym, everything I could do. . . . and by three months I was walking and no one could even notice a limp. And I went back to his office and he was shocked. Again another medical doctor, one of the best at what he does in the entire world, humbled, mystified, blown away.

He asked what I had done, and I told him, all of my natural healing programs. And I could see him rolling his eyes. He even yelled, THIS IS IMPOSSIBLE! His circuit boards were overloading, medical meltdown. He was so focused on being Dr. Frankenstein, cutting dead body parts out of one person and sewing them into another. He, like all of my other medical doctors, was so focused on his surgical procedure that he had never bothered to venture outside the medical mindset to see what might be another possible way that you could heal your body. He said to me, "Is this possible?"

I learned from my three traumatic scenarios, my deformed heart, my burnt-off hand and my torn-apart knee, that your body has some kind of blueprint or schematic of what perfect health is, and if you want to heal yourself all you have to do is get out of its way and let that happen. All you have to do is to stop doing whatever it is that is killing you or making you sick, and begin doing what will heal you. Why were the doctors wrong? (see The Faulty Mathematics of Medicine on page 44)

The bottom line: I have intensive and life-changing personal experience with my programs in this book. I also have positive healing results. If the medical doctors were right and my programs didn't work, I would have no hand, be crippled and, yeah, I would have DIED 30 YEARS AGO!

This also backs up the fact that I never asked a patient or reader to do anything that I haven't done myself a hundred times, and quite possibly a thousand. And I have gone deeper, farther, and with more intensity that I ever asked any patient to go.

MY EDUCATION AND TRAINING
WITH NATURAL HEALING AND HERBAL MEDICINE

Obviously my first (but *informal*) education was my three year experience in healing myself of a life-threatening disease and numerous supposed *incurable* injuries. After I healed myself, almost immediately the news spread, and sick relatives, friends and strangers literally crawled out of the woodwork asking me how I did it and what I thought would help them with not only their heart disease but also their cancer, diabetes, arthritis, neurological diseases, warts, *everything!* Personally looking back I have to laugh because I actually thought that I had only developed a detailed intensive program for healing deformed hearts. I never actually thought about what would happen if someone followed the same program for, say, cancer.

The knocks were coming on my door, and I remember thinking, well, it can't hurt them. Over the next few years I was astounded at the vast number of people with almost every different disease imaginable that were not just helped, but had actual healing miracles with my intensive *deformed heart and heart valve* natural healing program. I quickly learned that the healing power of living the fundamentals of good health were NOT disease specific and the programs I created successfully healed all diseases.

At this point in my life I decided that I wanted some *specific* education in Natural Healing and Herbal Medicine. I had taken numerous formal classes in pre-med courses from Psychology 101 to Anatomy and Physiology but I could see that they were all leading me towards the exact system of medicine that killed my parents, my short-lived friend in the hospital, and almost me. This would not do.

Therefore I decided to take courses in alternative medicine which were few and far between in those days, and also to just go and bother, hang around, intern, apprentice and absorb what I could from the great natural healing and herbal gurus of the day. My persistence and tough nature helped me gain entrance to some places and people that were considered unapproachable.

MY SELF-EDUCATION, AND MY RECOGNIZED CERTIFICATIONS AND DIPLOMAS

As a kid I grew up in a rural town with lots of truck farms. I sold seeds and had a vegetable garden every year. I worked on two farms.

Besides the hundred billion or so hours I spent in health food stores, co-ops and herbal stores researching and trying every product, I also worked in a co-op and behind the counter in an herbal pharmacy.

- **I followed a man named Paavo Airola around, the great European Naturopath, like a shadow. Wherever he spoke, I went. I bothered and pestered him with thousands of questions and picked up everything I could before he died.**

- I went to every health convention and expo that existed in those days for not only information but also to see who was who for my next teachers.

- I trained in nutrition and graduated with a degree in nutrition under Dr. Kurt Donsbach, the great nutritionist now heading Hospital Santa Monica in Mexico.

- I spent two years at UCLA auditing classes. I studied in their bio-med library on my own naturally designed curriculum of medical/natural healing. I think it would have been cheaper to pay tuition in the university than what I ended up paying to park my car at the hospital every day.

- I apprenticed with 2 chiropractors in trade for my knowledge, one a great Palmer graduate and another an old vegan eclectic doctor who had practiced in Hollywood, California since 1919.

- I am certified in 8 different styles of bodywork including Shiatsu, Applied Kinesology, Deep Tissue Restructuring, and trained extensively for years in Polarity Therapy with Dr. Rocannon MacGregor.

- I am certified in numerous systems of parapsychology, including Neuro-Linguistic Programming and Rebirthing.

- I received my teacher's certification in Hatha Yoga (Integral).

- I spent 22 years actively in the martial arts, earning 3 Black Belts. I am proficient in 5 other styles.

- I interned with the Great Dr. Bernard Jensen, the famous nutritionist and natural healer, author of over 500 books, and graduated from his school with 3 degrees and a truckload of common sense.

- I apprenticed with the late, great Dr John Ray Christopher, America's greatest herbalist of the last century. EVERYONE who is an herbalist today has borrowed material from this man. I studied directly under this great healer and he awarded me degrees as an Herbalist, a Master Herbalist, an Herbal Pharmacist, and eventually I received a Doctor of Herbology from his school. Dr. Christopher personally asked me to teach for him at his School of Natural Healing in Utah where I taught with him up until his death and then as the senior professor for many years for his family.

As part of what I consider my education I taught herbal medicine every summer for 15 years in Great Britain, France and Spain. I taught at Cambridge University in Cambridge, England, Trinity Medical College in Dublin, Ireland, and at natural healing schools, herbal colleges and health retreats. In Europe and America I have over 1,000 clinically practicing graduates. With many I have created their clinical protocols.

I am a founding member of the British Herbal Practitioners Association and have participated with various British Herbal Colleges to consolidate curriculums and assure continued presence in the EEC.

I have had what I consider the best training in Natural Healing and Herbal Medicine. I studied, trained, interned and apprenticed with people who I think were the best natural healers and herbal doctors of the time. Almost all of my training was clinical training, which I believe is the best.

MY CLINICAL EXPERIENCE
USING NATURAL HEALING AND HERBAL MEDICINE

I began my first clinic in New York State in the early 1970's. I moved to Southern California and continued my clinics in Hollywood, North Hollywood, Pacific Palisades, Santa Monica and Malibu, California. **My clinics were open spanning three decades, over 20 years, with over 20,000 patient visits in this country and abroad.**

In the last decade of my clinical practice I specialized in degenerative and life-threatening diseases. Especially the ones medicine says are incurable, like Cancer, AIDS, Heart Disease, Arthritis, Diabetes, Liver and Kidney failure, Alzheimer's Disease and other Neurological diseases. The news of my success with these patients and their life-threatening diseases spread. My clinical success became an embarrassment to the medical community, and my patients' thriving instead of dying became embarrassing living testimonials to the failure of modern medicine. I was arrested and my clinic was boarded up.

I consider this governmental action one of my greatest achievements, an award similar to that of my great teachers. (Dr. Jensen had many close calls with the law and Dr. Christopher was arrested and jailed on 6 occasions). I had done well, and so had my patients.

MY NATURAL HEALING AND HERBAL PROGRAMS
ARE SIMPLE AND MAKE GOOD COMMON SENSE

I admit, I am a very robust, larger than life, outspoken, radical, revolutionary, visionary, intense, butt-kicking, passionate, opinionated, dynamic, loud, aggressive, and even violent Natural Healing Evangelist.

Many people have many problems with me, my mannerisms and my methods.

BUT, no one has ever said my programs don't work. In fact, just the opposite. And no one has ever said my programs don't make good common sense, because they all do.

Just read this book. Nothing in it is rocket science, and I hardly use any twenty dollar words. It is basic, fundamental, simple and foundational Natural Healing and Herbal Medicine.

I AM STILL ALIVE

This is in response to my comment and warning on books from dead authors.

WHAT I KNOW

If you are looking for a person who knows the many names of the many phytochemicals in herbs, can identify the many medicinal herbs in the woods or has the deepest knowledge of botany, I am NOT this person.

If you're looking for a man who KNOWS how to:

**Help people heal themselves
of any disease and any sickness.**

**Help people create powerful health
and to stay healthy.**

And know how to do this all NATURALLY!
I am your man.

DR. SCHULZE'S CLINICAL CHARTS AND AFFIRMATIONS

The following charts and quotes are what I used to wake up, educate, illuminate and enlighten the thousands of patients and students that walked through the doors of my clinic.

First and foremost I needed to wake my patients up to let them know that they were not entering just *another* doctor's office. Sick people usually wander from doctor to doctor like zombies, hoping that the next doctor they see will be the one with the *magic pill* that will heal their disease. This is the common thought pattern of most people whether they are going to medical doctors *or* natural doctors. Find the magic pill.

This is simply because the *business of medicine* has indoctrinated and brainwashed all of us since we were young children in the idea of *finding* a cure. Just the word "finding" implies looking outside yourself for the answer. We were all taught that healing is a matter of *finding* the right cure for your particular disease and that usually this cure would be a *chemical* called a *drug* and this drug would either be in the form of a *pill* or an *injection*. My patients were really no different than people who go to medical doctors except that they were looking for a *natural drug* or a *natural pill* or a *natural injection* to cure their disease. Often they were investigating natural means only because the medical drugs and pills had already failed them but in any case, same medical mentality. The bottom line is that they were looking for a *natural* pill cure.

So immediately I had to do something to throw them. This probably comes from my background in Ju Jitsu. I had to stop them right away, before they even entered my clinic, and help them understand that if they entered my clinic door, they would no longer be searching for that pill cure for their dis-ease, whether chemical or natural. That they would no longer be trying to *find* a cure. That instead they would be taking *RESPONSIBILITY* for <u>themselves</u> *and* <u>their disease</u> from this moment on.

So, hung on the *outside* of my clinic door (so they could run away at the last minute and save themselves the embarrassment of looking foolish) I had a sign stating:

"Everyone is looking for a good doctor. <u>I am looking for great patients</u>."

This is not just a matter of semantics or playing tricks with words.
<u>Responsibility is the</u> **FOUNDATION** of Natural Healing

It is what sets Natural healing apart from every other type of healing system there is, medical and alternative. The fact that my door sign says that I am looking for great patients implies *their active role* in the healing of *their* disease. My sign would immediately trigger a different thought process from a different perspective. Now they would begin to see their healing as a journey, an adventure, a trip to hell and back, whatever, but definitely **NOT** a pill.

My absolute focus then and now is to help people to heal *themselves*. Therefore I needed to educate my patients to understand what Natural Healing is, how it is different than other forms of healing and medicine, and most importantly *their responsibility* in this healing process. I knew that the more I could educate them, and keep them awake and conscious, <u>the better chance they would have at healing their diseases.</u>

Once they came through my clinic door, looking a little stunned and maybe a little afraid, they would then see the first sign *inside* of my clinic, which read:

"<u>Healing Your Disease and Getting Well is Easy.</u> All you have to do is <u>STOP</u> doing the things that made you sick in the first place and <u>START</u> new healthy habits that will create a powerful healing."

If my new patient hadn't got it yet from the sign on the *outside* of the front door, which nobody did, I felt it necessary to hit them again, before they could catch their breath (more martial arts I guess). So again, I wanted to remind them that this is **NOT** a medical doctor's office, that I am **NOT** a medical doctor and, most importantly, that I was **NOT** going to *bullshit* them into thinking that their disease could be healed with a few drugs and maybe a little surgery or radiation. I did **NOT** want them fantasizing that they could be healed with no participation, no lifestyle changes, no upsetting their usual routine, no healthy living, no nutritional support and no cleansing or detoxification; just live life like you usually do, relax, sit back, and let me pretend I am God and I will heal you.

I wanted them to know from their first second in my clinic that *they were going to do all the work.* Sure, I'm human and so there is part of me that wishes that I was Jesus and could wave my hand over someone's face and heal all their diseases, especially the children, but I'm not and I can't, **so it's time to get to work!**

THE FIRST FIVE MINUTES
IN DR. SCHULZE'S CLINIC

First off you must understand that with the vast majority of patients that came to see me in my clinic, I wasn't their first choice. In fact I was usually their last-ditch, desperate attempt to heal themselves before undergoing some treatment or surgery that was more frightening, painful and potentially lethal, than their disease.

My staff would always instruct them to bring every single piece of paper that they had acquired during their **disease journey.** Because most of my new patients had already been to numerous medical doctors, maybe even in the hospital, and had numerous tests done. They would come in with an armful or even a boxful of charts, x-rays, ultrasounds, biopsy reports, blood and urine tests and literally handfuls of papers held together by paper clips or rubber bands.

As I mentioned earlier my new patients had almost always gone to just about every natural healer and alternative medicine doctor in town. This is simply because I had a reputation to be the Natural Doctor from Hell, Dirty Harry, the guy no one wants to use but when the shit hits the fan you call him. Some patients referred to me as Adolph because of my German decent and my natural Gestapo tactics. But regardless of what they had heard about me, they had also heard the rumor that when undergoing my treatment, they were going to be forced to do what turned out to be the hardest thing to do that they had ever done in their life . . . . *change*.

Who they are now is Cancer, Heart Disease, AIDS, Parkinson's or Alzheimer's Disease, and I am going to help them through a metamorphosis into a new life, a new healthy body mind and spirit, and in a way, who they were when they walked through my clinic door **has to DIE**, and be reborn. That's right, they were either going to die from their disease that was killing them or die because they had to change into a totally new person, physically, emotionally and spiritually. Talk about being between a rock and a hard place. I would have felt sorry for them except that I have been in that place on numerous occasions myself with my own healing journey. And I wouldn't want to take that wonderful healing experience away from anybody, even if I could. So any way you look at it, *they were dead!*

So back to the medical paperwork: under the opposite arm was a huge folder of natural doctor tests like hair analysis reports, cytotoxic blood analysis, aura scans, parasite and Candida albicans reports, radionics readings, psychic and astrological readings, advice from channels and past life regressionists and various other reports, charts and graphs from alternative testing and diagnosis machines that are constantly surfacing in the natural medicine world. So on top of having one or more standard medical disease they also were proven by alternative testing to be hypoglycemic, of course had Candida albicans overgrowth, were bipolar, mildly dyslexic, manic depressive, abused by their parents, toxic, they're illeocecal valve was stuck open (or was it closed?), and also had a complex synergy of eating disorders including anorexia, bulimia, excessive/compulsive overeater and undereater and probably had a very traumatic past life too.

Again I am not making fun of any medical or alternative diagnosis, prognosis, reports, tests and findings. I am saying that in natural healing virtually none of it was necessary. I am bored with the sick and diseased past. I don't even want to know about it much less talk about it. This is simply because Natural Healing is the healing science of creating the future by creating the most powerful and positive healing lifestyle and environment surrounding the patient, that is literally so healthy that their body responds by healing their disease. As an example, when a person removes their physical, emotional and spiritual abuse which can be anything from hot dogs and cigarettes to constipation and self-hatred, and then adds a few health promoting programs to their life such as fresh juice, routine cleansing and detoxification and a positive self image, presto, the human body always responds by healing itself. It's that simple. If the patient doesn't respond at all or not enough, then it is just a matter of finding more health-destroying bad habits to remove and adding more health-promoting programs. I would always eventually tell my patients that their disease will go away and they will be healthy and strong somewhere between drinking one glass of fresh organic apple juice and a 20-year intensive cleansing program. The only way to find out what it's going to take is to get started.

So I would ask them for all of their papers, charts, reports and test results and I would study them for only a few minutes. Then I would ask them if they were willing to do anything to get well and almost everyone's first answer was yes.

If you ask most people if they would like a brand new Mercedes Benz automobile their first answer is usually YES! But then when the average person sees what the actual cost is, the thousand dollar auto payments and insurance bills, well all of a sudden that rusty old clunker doesn't look so bad after all. My point is almost everyone says that they are willing to do anything to get well when they are sick, but when they heard that my natural healing program wasn't just a matter of swallowing some new herbal magic bullet pill, well . . . . . now their disease wasn't really that bad after all. They can live with a few aches and pains, maybe even get that kidney transplant. After all there is such a thing as the quality of life and to some people giving up their favorite candy bar, well that's just taking things a little bit too far.

So here I am sitting with my new patient and their thousands of dollars worth of papers and I NOW HAD TO GET THEIR ATTENTION, I HAD TO SAVE THEIR LIFE, so with each new patient I would then proceed to throw away all of their years of paperwork, paperwork that proved beyond a shadow of a doubt that they were really screwed up, sick, diseased and dying, INTO A BIG BLACK TRASH BIN that I kept in my examination room. This was not because any or all of the test reports and results were invalid, it was because **I was about to show them a whole new world of health and healing that was literally beyond their imaginations.**

In the meantime this act with my trash bin didn't go unnoticed. In fact, just the opposite, it would cause involuntary leaps, jerks, muscle spasms, yelling, screaming, crying, swearing, drooling and dribbling and on many occasions I was slapped or punched (thank God again for my practice of the Martial Arts). The next move was that people would often fall to the floor on their hands and knees and desperately try to grasp the numerous papers, pictures and charts that were all getting mixed up and out of order and almost unconsciously try to sort them out and get them all back into order. Now as they were grabbing them I would start ripping them up, which always caused a secondary panic of them trying to salvage what they could from this obvious madman. Often at this moment they would be yelling at me that all of this paperwork cost them tens of thousands of dollars and that they would sue me. At some point this confrontation would literally develop into rolling and wrestling around the floor until they were exhausted.

In many instances patients that had degenerative nerve diseases, where medical doctors said that they would never talk again (and their partner or relative confirmed that they actually hadn't spoke in years), well, the mute patient actually screamed and called me a dirty bastard, son of a bitch or some other colorful name. Many times those in wheelchairs who were crippled walked instantly, actually ran. So for some the healing miracle had already begun, instantly, but for all of them they would eventually see that I was going to win, and I almost always did, and this was now, **the beginning of their healing journey. I could now see in their tearful and glazed eyes that they knew something wonderful was about to happen.** In fact many told me months later that they felt more alive in that few seconds after our confrontation than they had in the previous years with all their doctors rolled up into one.

From this moment on they knew that I was different than any doctor they had gone to before. They also knew that we were now going to stop focusing on their disease, their illness, their tumor, their malignancy, their nerve damage, their dying . . . . . and shift our focus to their

LIVING!

And most importantly we are going to, as the sign said, "STOP **doing the things that made them sick in the first place and** START **new healthy habits that will create powerful health".**

MY CLINICAL CHARTS AND HANDOUTS

After a year or so in practice I obviously found myself having to repeat over and over certain natural healing fundamentals and programs to the point that if I had to explain them one more time I think I would have exploded. This was a great awareness for me because I realized that if I had to repeat these same things to every patient, over and over and over . . . THESE MUST BE VERY IMPORTANT FUNDAMENTALS OF HEALTH AND HEALING.

Consequently many of the following charts were made not just so I wouldn't explode, but also to help my patients understand what Natural Healing is, how it works and how they can best succeed at it. Many of the quotes were to remind them how simple natural healing is and who is in charge, *their* Responsibility.

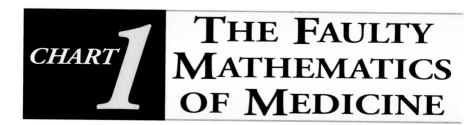

CHART 1 — THE FAULTY MATHEMATICS OF MEDICINE

This was a handout that I gave my patients on their first visit. The reason why is simple: they had lost their souls to their disease. They were no longer Mary Jones or Bob Smith, they were now the sum total of their tests. They were Mrs. A-lateral sclerosis or Mr. Hodgkin's disease.

They had lost sight of all the wonderful things about life and about themselves. They were so focused on what was wrong they missed all the things that were right. They had no vision of the future except disease, doctors and death. They were no longer able to laugh, only to cry. They were no longer able to see the light, only the darkness. They had no strength, only fear, and they had lost their love and were filled with rage and hate. They were very sick.

My first job before they could begin to heal themselves was to get them to *believe* in the possibility that they could heal themselves.

So once I got them to stop crying and shaking, or hitting me, and begin to breathe, I would then give them my first chart, **The Faulty Mathematics of Medicine.**

The main purpose of this chart is to show the patient that all of the doctors that they have seen, especially the medical doctors, were working with a faulty mathematical equation. Although their diagnosis (the name of their disease defined by the sum total of their symptoms) may be somewhat correct, what we could work to invalidate was the doctors' Prognosis (their supposed future), or the supposed *normal* progression of their *disease*. What I said to them and what I am saying to you is that all medical Prognoses are just a guess of the future. They are not set in stone, THEY ARE NOT THE ABSOLUTE FUTURE! They are pretty accurate guesses based on the usual outcome of the *AVERAGE* person who has this particular disease, but they are NOT absolute.

I would explain to them that if they continued to be *average*, that they could probably expect everything that the medical doctor said will happen will come true. But what if they chose to <u>NOT</u> be the *Average American?* Well, this *throws off this entire mathematical equation.* As you can see in my chart, a medical doctor diagnoses you with the name of a disease that is the closest pick from your group of symptoms. They have probably backed this up with blood tests, x-rays, MRI's, whatever. Medical doctors are pretty good at this and pretty accurate.

But here is where they go wrong: they make an *assumption* that you are the Average American and therefore they will give you a Prognosis (you will be dead in a month). <u>Any first year science or math student will tell you that an *assumption* is *the mother of all screw-ups*.</u> See, the medical doctors are *assuming* that you are the Average American, and you probably are. **But what if you decided NOT to continue to be the Average American? To Change!** What if you decided to be a Non-Average American. <u>Well, then this same first year science or math student would flatly tell you that the medical equation is now invalid because one of the constants had changed.</u>

<u>The bottom line is what I saw in my clinic, and was able to consistently repeat with thousands of patients, is that if my patients were willing to change, and not live like the Average American, and chose to live a healthier life by creating a healthy lifestyle, that their medical Prognosis was not only incorrect, it was bullshit!</u> So instead of dying in 30 days, or whatever the medical doctor said was going to happen, **IT DID NOT HAPPEN! What DID happen is that my patients' diseases went into remission, went away, disappeared, poof, gone, and they went on to live long healthy lives, often outliving the medical doctors who gave them the death sentence in the first place.**

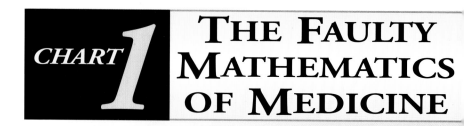

CHART 1 — THE FAULTY MATHEMATICS OF MEDICINE

What is the _missing factor_ in this medical equation?

$$D + M? = P$$

DIAGNOSIS

The _name_ a doctor puts on your particular group of symptoms that they believe is your _dis-ease_.

+ THE MISSING FACTOR

(Are you the average American?)

= PROGNOSIS

Prediction of the course and end of a disease, and the _estimate_ of your chance for recovery.

THE MISSING FACTOR is that the doctor believes you are the Average American. Let's take a look at the Average American's lifestyle:

- They eat a low nutrition, high fat and sugar food program, a diet high in over-processed, nutritionally depleted food.

- They consume 300 soft drinks, 170 pounds of white refined sugar, 400 candy bars and 500 doughnuts a year, and will eat over 12 entire 3,000 pound cows, 6 whole pigs, 3,000 chickens and other birds and another 3,000 assorted fish and sea creatures and over 30,000 quarts of milk in their lifetime and try to pass all of this through their digestive system and bloodstream.

- They will have an average of 2 - 4 bowel movements a week, coming up 70,000 bowel movements short in their lifetime, definitely having diverticulosis and digestive and elimination problems.

- They will get very little exercise, if any, be 25 pounds or more overweight, have hypercholesterolemia with an average level of 200 and have high blood pressure.

- They take over 30,000 aspirin and assorted other pain killers in their lifetime along with over 20,000 over the counter and prescription drugs and over 2,000 gallons of alcohol.

- The average American has a negative self-image, and experiences recurring bouts of depression and anxiety. The Average American is physically, emotionally and spiritually sick. Therefore, the doctor's prognosis of their disease is probably statistically correct.

ON THE CONTRARY, if you live an above average lifestyle, a healthy lifestyle, doctors will know little or nothing about how your body will react and recover from disease or your healing potential. You can expect to have medical miracles happen like Dr. Schulze's heart, hand, knee and all of his patients.

One reason they are pretty accurate is books like the Merck Manual, published by the drug company Merck, Sharpe and Dome. This book is compiled and written by a team of the most educated and *"best in their field"* medical doctors from all over the world, and is on the desk of EVERY medical doctor in America. It is considered to be the greatest and most accurate book of Diagnosis and Prognosis in common use covering thousands of different diseases, their numerous symptoms and the team consensus of what the best therapeutic protocols are.

But all of this knowledge doesn't mean squat *if you change* a parameter in the equation, the key words being, If <u>YOU</u> Change!

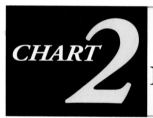

CHART 2

THE DIFFERENCE BETWEEN NATURAL HEALING AND MEDICAL INTERVENTION

Now that I got my patient to realize that they didn't have to succumb to their medical doctor's prognosis, I used my next chart to begin to show them some of the fundamental differences between Natural Healing and Medicine. Understanding these differences would help my patients develop what I called a Natural Healing *filter* in their brain. In the same way as in the very beginning of this book I gave you tips on how to judge the validity of a book by its author, this chart helped my patients from falling astray when trying to determine whether or not a food, therapeutic treatment or even an emotion was a part of natural healing or medicine.

	NATURAL HEALING	MEDICAL INTERVENTION
FOCUS	To **Create** a Healthy Person	To **Destroy**, Kill or Cure a Disease
METHOD OF TREATMENT	Setting up a proper living *environment* so our body can heal itself. This is done through changes in our Food Program, Elimination, Movement, Emotions and Lifestyle. **Assistance**	Attacking, Killing and Removing disease using drugs and surgery. Altering or removing malfunctioning parts or organs. (ex. coronary bypass surgery, appendectomy, mastectomy.) **Intervention**
THERAPEUTIC PRODUCTS	**Products of Nature** Wholesome Fruits, Vegetables, Grains, Seeds, Sprouts, Nuts, Herbs, Concentrated whole food supplements such as my SuperFood. **NO Side Effects**	**Man Made Products** Isolated Drugs made from petro-chemicals, animal waste and toxic elements. Man made vitamin and mineral pills. **MANY Side Effects including Iatrogenic DEATH**
THERAPEUTIC MODALITIES	Vegetarian (Vegan) Food Programs, Cleansing and Detoxification Routines, Exercise and Movement, Bodywork, Hydrotherapy, Emotional Healing, and **changes in the way we <u>live,</u> <u>work,</u> <u>play</u> and <u>relate.</u>**	Surgery, Radiation, Toxic Chemotherapy, Stimulant, Sedative and Suppressive drugs, Carnivore DIEtetics, Dialysis, Colostomies, **changes in one's <u>lifestyle</u> and <u>habits</u> are rarely discussed.**
EMOTIONS	**Positive Attitude** Excitement, Strength, Trust in God and Nature, Love, Laughter, Empowerment.	**Negative Attitude** Coping, Anxiety, Fear, Weakness, Depression, Being out of Control, Our life is in someone else's hands.
RESPONSIBILITY	We have **created** our current health level and therefore we can change it and heal ourself. Being in **control.**	I "caught" this disease. I am an unlucky **victim.** Doctor/God, please heal me.

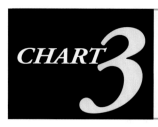

THE FUNDAMENTAL CATEGORIES THAT DETERMINE YOUR LEVEL OF HEALTH

Your current level of health is a perfect reflection of how your body, mind and spirit is responding to the <u>environment</u> and <u>lifestyle</u> you have created for yourself.

INTAKE:	The quality of the air we breathe, the liquid we drink and the food we eat.
ELIMINATION:	The function and efficiency of our organs designed to remove and expel waste.
MOVEMENT AND CIRCULATION:	The ways we move our body to keep it toned, flexible, with good circulation.
LIFESTYLE:	How we live, work and play.
EMOTIONS AND SPIRIT:	Do we have positive healing or negative destructive emotional and spiritual habits?
INHERITED CONSTITUTION:	Your physical, emotional and spiritual constitution inherited from your parents, your genetics and what you choose to do about it.

These factors all determine...
YOUR CURRENT LEVEL OF HEALTH.
Your entire body totally rebuilds itself in less than 2 years!!!

98% in less than 1 year. A new brain in 1 year, blood in 4 months, skeleton in 3 months, DNA in 2 months, liver in 6 weeks, skin in 1 month and stomach lining in 5 days!!!!!

WHY ARE YOU STILL CREATING THE SAME BODY???

THE FOUNDATIONS OF NATURAL HEALING
BY DR. RICHARD SCHULZE

RESPONSIBILITY

"The first fundamental principle of Natural Healing is Responsibility.
Responsibility literally means, *the ability to respond.*
This means taking charge of your life and being Responsible for
EVERYTHING that goes in and out of your body, mind and spirit."

"I have seen a lot of strange things in my life, but I've never seen a farmer
plant strawberries and have corn come up instead. You reap what you sow.
Tomorrow is what you DO and BELIEVE Today!"

SIMPLICITY

"Healing Disease and Getting Well is very simple and easy.
All you have to do is . . .

STOP what you did that made you sick in the first place . . . and
START new habits that will heal you and create vibrant health.
And the miracle happens . . ."

"Complex, complicated and intricate programs feed the ego of the
doctor and are impossible for the patient to live with. It's the simple
programs that got my patients well.
Keep it simple. If it's too complicated, simplify it . . . or throw it out."

CHANGE

Your body has a blueprint, a schematic, of what perfect health is
and it's constantly trying to achieve this goal for you.

"There are NO Incurable diseases, NONE.
Your body can heal itself of ANY disease and ANY Illness
and you can create a healthy, energetic, vibrant and amazing life.
All you have to do is Change."

PREFACE
TO MY 20 STEPS

Most of you know that a medical doctor said that I'd be dead thirty years ago, but instead I'm healthier now than I was then. In order to achieve all of my personal healing miracles and then help literally tens of thousands of patients and students create all of their healing miracles, I developed a set of disciplines, exercise, tips—whatever you want to call them—to live by. These tips saved my life. And then they saved the lives of thousands and thousands of my patients all around the world.

Some of these tips are pretty easy, and you might be doing some of them already. Better yet, you might be doing them every day. Others, well, they might take a lifetime to master. All I can tell you is that each one of them is powerfully life-changing, and if you dare to include all of them in your life, you will live the life that you've only dreamed is possible, an amazingly healthful, vibrant, truthful, joyous and loving life. This kind of life will no longer be just a dream or a hope, but it will become a reality for you. These twenty steps may take twenty years to master, but you could actually add twenty years to your life. Isn't that worth it? Remember what I said on page 38 of this book— that getting well is easy. All you have to do is stop doing what it was that made you sick, and start living new and healthy ways that will heal you. Start adding healthy programs to your life that will raise your level of health so high that all disease will be destroyed. It will run right out of your body. So let's get started.

Dr. Richard Schulze

DR. SCHULZE
QUOTE:

"The healing journey that you are about to embark on IS A GIFT, a BLESSING, not a burden or a hardship.

It is the beginning of your greatest adventure *inward,* to discover and create a new life, to create a NEW YOU!"

1 CHAPTER ONE

PURE WATER

Drink at least one quart of pure water every day.

WHY SHOULD I?

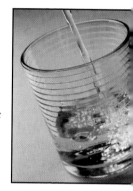

Liquid is what the vast majority of you is made out of. You are a big water balloon. Take away the water in your body and all that's left is just a few pounds of bones and ash. Did you ever see someone's ashes after cremation? It's a little pot of bone chunks and ash. That's you without water. From Constipation, to High Blood Pressure, from Kidney and Liver disease to Colds and Cancer, your body is assisted in healing ALL diseases IMMEDIATELY just by drinking more water every day.

FACTS

- Your body is 85% liquid, your brain alone is 75% liquid.

- You lose about a quart of water a day just by breathing.

- Drinking more water REDUCES your risk of developing cancer and heart disease.

- Pure water flushes waste, poisons and toxins from your entire system.

- Chlorination, the most widely used method of killing bacteria in water, is known to produce powerful carcinogenic residues, including Dioxin. Studies have shown that the risk of bladder cancer is doubled if you drink chlorine-treated water. Chlorination also destroys Vitamin E in the body, which can lead to heart problems, and has been linked to clogged arteries.

HOW TO DO IT?

By beginning to drink more pure water every day, you assist your body in building the fluids it needs to survive and thrive, like blood and lymphatic fluid. You also assist your body to eliminate waste and toxins. The only catch is that you have to drink PURE water and not water that contains anything that will hurt you.

Since water is considered the universal solvent, it tends to attract and absorb many things that it comes in contact with. Since the water table on earth is below the ground, things also tend to settle there. Because of this most scientists agree that the entire world's water source is polluted with industrial chemicals. I know that is hard to believe but many very toxic and poisonous industrial pollutants are now found in water samples taken on the entire earth.

Cleaning up the world's water supply is another issue. What I am concerned with in the scope of this book is you getting more pure water into your body.

I hope I don't have to convince you that any municipal tap water is unfit to drink. C'mon. Added chlorine and other disinfectants, added fluoride made from waste aluminum, supposed *acceptable* levels of the industrial pollutants, agricultural pollutants, insecticides and pesticides. All the chemical *stuff* that's oozed and leaked from manufacturing for the past hundred and fifty years all over the world. I don't care where you live or what bull your local water company says, even well water has PCBs in it and other industrial contaminants well-known to cause cancer and 100 other diseases. So the day of pure water from the ground is over.

So the best water for you to drink is water that is purified.

Distilled water may be the cleanest water available. It also happens to be the best for cleansing and detoxifying the body. This is simply because it is very EMPTY water and wants to dissolve and attract impurities out of your body. It also happens to be the best water to use for making herbal tea because it will dissolve and accept more of the phytochemicals from the plant and therefore make a stronger herbal tea. You can buy a water distiller and make distilled water yourself. They can cost a few hundred to a few thousand dollars and take a little bit of time to operate and clean but for the most serious, this is a great way to go.

Reverse Osmosis runs neck and neck with distilled water. In fact, I have seen some reverse osmosis equipment that actually makes cleaner and more empty water down to lower microns of contaminants than distilled water. These systems cost a few hundred to a thousand dollars and hook up right under your sink and you only have to replace parts once a year with no regular maintenance.

Ceramic Water filters also remove literally everything from water and have become more and more popular recently. I have tested many and they all are great.

Simple charcoal water filters are also extremely effective at removing almost all poisons and most contaminants from water.

My great aunt Hattie outlived all of my other relatives in the entire family. She didn't do anything special or different than any other family members EXCEPT, she boiled all of her water. She had a ritual every day and boiled all of her water and I remember as a young child she warned me with a very stern look on her face, "never trust anything that comes out of a tap, always boil it before you drink it". She was right.

The bottom line: just do the best you can and drink chemical-free and bacteria-free water. This is the first step in getting well—drinking clean, pure water. I don't really care how you clean it or purify it and I am never going to get into an argument defending one type of water to another. Just do it. Water is the universal solvent. It dissolves waste in your body and flushes you clean. It replenishes what you are made out of and lubricates you. Start drinking at least one quart of pure water every day.

DR. SCHULZE

QUOTE: "Your body has the ability to completely heal itself of any disease . . .

All it needs is your assistance."

2 CHAPTER TWO

FRESH JUICE

Drink one quart of fresh juice every day.

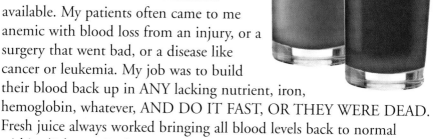

WHY SHOULD I?

Fresh juice is the most powerful natural blood builder and blood transfusion available. My patients often came to me anemic with blood loss from an injury, or a surgery that went bad, or a disease like cancer or leukemia. My job was to build their blood back up in ANY lacking nutrient, iron, hemoglobin, whatever, AND DO IT FAST, OR THEY WERE DEAD. Fresh juice always worked bringing all blood levels back to normal within 48 hours. It always worked, 100% of the time.

FACTS

- Fresh Juice is the fastest and most natural way to build healthy and powerful blood.

- The concentrated amount of vitamins, minerals, enzymes and other life-giving nutrients in juice assimilates very easily and quickly into your blood. The nutrients in juice can even be assimilated in your mouth and be into your cells, literally in seconds, traveling to every organ and cell in your body *fast.*

- I have personally revived and brought dying patients back to life with a glass of juice.

- Fresh juice naturally detoxifies your body. It does this by stimulating many elimination organs like your Liver, Gall Bladder, Kidneys and Intestines to eliminate more waste. It also cleanses, detoxifies and heals these organs too.

- Fresh Fruit and Vegetable Juice is naturally very alkalinizing, cleansing and detoxifying to your blood. It facilitates the phagocytosis, or the speed and ability of your white blood cells, like macrophages, to clean your blood and tissues of bacteria, virus, fungus, and many harmful pathogenic micro-organisms, even malignant cancer cells.

HOW TO DO IT?
IN MY CLINIC

In my clinic, especially during my last ten years of practice, I spent most of my time helping patients with degenerative diseases. These are the diseases that modern medicine calls incurable, like Cancer, AIDS, Degenerative Artery Disease, Alzheimer's Disease, Diabetes, Arthritis, most Liver and Kidney Disease, the neurological diseases like Parkinson's and A-Lateral Sclerosis, etc...

So when I saw a patient on the first visit I would explain to them that a prerequisite for them to be allowed to return for their second visit was that they had to buy a juicer, AND BEGIN TO USE IT before they came in for their second visit. No juicer and I would fire them, and they would not be allowed to see me until they got their juicer. This act alone should impress upon you the importance of making and drinking fresh juice every day, especially if you are sick.

Some patients would come back for their second visit with excuses but not a juicer. Many of my staff remember me literally throwing patients right out the front door of my clinic, by the back of their neck. Yes, even the gray-haired old grannies. If you don't have the money, sell something. Sell your television. Sell your furniture and sit on the floor. Sell your car and walk. Sell your clothes. But don't live another day without a juicer.

WHAT KIND OF JUICER IS THE BEST?

What kind, you ask? I own them all. Try them all out and see which one you like best. Basically I find the centrifugal juicers that don't eject pulp to be a pain in the butt because you have to stop juicing and open them constantly and clean them out. So I don't advise those.

One great juicer that has lasted me 30 years now is my Champion. This great juicer is made so tough and durable that your grandchildren will inherit it. I have used this juicer making juice daily for 30 students on a juice fast for an entire week on numerous occasions. It got so hot you couldn't touch the motor, but it kept on juicing. They cost about $300.00 (about 20 minutes in the hospital).

The slower operating Green Power or Green Life type juicers definitely get more juice out of dryer things like carrots, roots and greens, and I believe the juice is better quality. But these juicers don't do juicy fruits very well and are a little more difficult to clean. The best is to have a Champion for your juicy fruits and vegetables and a Green Power for your dryer fruits and vegetables. But if you can only have one, I would choose the Champion, which also makes raw nut butters and my favorite, fresh frozen fruit fake ice cream. (Hint, use frozen bananas without the peel as the base and then put any other frozen fruit through the Champion, but alternating with bananas.)

No one will argue that the Norwalk Juicer, named after the awesome old natural healer Norman Walker, is the best. There are others modeled after the Norwalk juicer, like the K & K juicer, which are also great. This type of juicer grates the substance to be juiced first, and then presses it hydraulically. There is no doubt that this type of juicer gets more essential nutrients out of the material juiced and is better. The cost of this type of juicer is about $1,000.00 to $2,000.00.

The Juiceman juicers aren't in the high quality category as the above juicers, but they work just fine. I like Jay's energy and passion for juice and I think they even give you a video on how to use it, some sample recipes and a 1-800-I can't figure it out phone number for the juicer-challenged. Juicers that are physically smaller than the Juiceman juicers with tiny motors often burn out when they meet their first tough carrot. They are a waste of money.

Some people say get a Vita-Mix which is like a high speed industrial blender. They say this blender makes *total* juice by liquifying fruits and vegetables with added water, and then drinking the liquid and the pulp. This might be more nutritious, but it gagged many of my patients. I love my vita-mix and use it for many things, from making raw soups to garlic spread, but it is not a juicer.

EXCUSES

Some people say, "Well, but what about the sugar in juice?" C'mon now. Don't let your big <u>but</u> get in the way of creating a new life. I had diabetics who healed their diabetes with juice fasting. For some of you, diluting your fresh juices with water will make them easier to digest and assimilate, and easier on your body's metabolism. I often dilute my juices with water.

Some people say, I can't find organic fruits or veggies so I don't want to juice. No doubt about it, organic fruits and vegetables have 4 to 10 times more nutrition in them, have no harmful agriculture chemical residues on them like pesticides and insecticides and support a clean earth. But don't stop if you can't get organic. Get the best produce you can and get started juicing.

IS JUICE REALLY NATURAL?

Some people say that juice isn't natural. Well, it isn't natural. By extracting the juice out of a fruit or vegetable—now we're making a very concentrated substance, a medicine, and this isn't truly natural. It is no longer in its natural state. But neither is the way we now live; neither is the way we have abused ourselves and our bodies for the past twenty or thirty years. Life as we live it is not natural anymore. We are bombarded on a daily basis with toxic chemicals in the food we eat, the air we breathe, and the liquid we drink. So we have already swung the pendulum too far in one direction of living a decadent life, a life that degenerates our body, ages us prematurely and creates disease. A life that kills a body designed to last 100, 200, 300?? years, in only 50 or 60 years. Now, what I am asking you is to swing that pendulum a little too far in the healthy direction, a little unnatural on the positive side—extracting juice out of fruits and vegetables. There's one thing I know: modern civilized life is not natural, so we have to swing that pendulum the other way and make juice and drink a quart a day. Juice will not only detoxify, cleanse and flush out your body, but it will give you nutrients that you cannot assimilate from just eating food. Therefore it is the perfect food for sick people who all have limited digestive and assimilation abilities.

ELIMINATE A FEW BAD DRINKS WHILE YOU ARE AT IT

Note: steps one and two are to drink a quart each of pure water and fresh juice every day. Try adding an additional quart of herbal tea.

At the same time I would like you to eliminate any liquids that you drink that are toxic or destructive to your body, like coffee, black tea or any beverage containing caffeine, soda pop and any carbonated beverage including carbonated water which is all pumped with carbon dioxide which is a waste product of the human body, and any alcoholic drinks. I am not saying that an occasional cup of coffee or a glass of wine ever killed anyone, but they have no place on a health-building program or as a routine maintenance beverage in your life. They are party foods only.

When I drive to work in the morning to the American Botanical Pharmacy, I pass two places about seven a.m. and both of them have lines of grumpy, anxious, miserable people standing outside waiting for their fix. One of them is a coffee shop and one of them is a cocaine drug house, and I don't see the difference, nor does your body. OK, one is legal, but they're both long lines of people shaking and waiting for their fix.

A FINAL NOTE

Never underestimate the power of fresh juices. Many internationally famous cancer clinics have each patient drink about 3 quarts of fresh juice a day. Even the American Cancer Society states that nutrients in fruit and vegetable juice REDUCE your risk of developing cancer and they recommend many servings a day.

DR. SCHULZE'S BLOOD BUILDER VEGETABLE JUICE RECIPE

This is the one that I took to the hospital that saved hundreds of my patients from death. The sooner you can drink it after pressing, the better.

> 8 ounces of organic Carrot Juice
> 5 ounces of organic Beet Root juice
> 2 ounces of organic Beet Greens juice
> 1 ounce of organic Wheat Grass juice

If you prefer using fruit, use Apple and Grape juice to clean your blood or any Grape, Blueberry, Blackberry, Raspberry, Cherry, Prune, and any purple, blue or dark red fruit you can get to build your blood.

HELP YOUR CHILDREN TO LOVE DRINKING JUICES TOO!

Often children who haven't had juice and had sodas and junk drinks will shy away from fresh juice, especially a glass of carrot juice. What I would do with my child patients is, first, get them personally involved with the juicing process. Most kids find this fun and entertaining, like a science project. Just watch their little fingers when the juicers are running and always keep them UNPLUGGED until you actually need to turn them on. Secondly, start them first on fresh apple juice, which almost every child loves. Then after a few days make 90% apple and 10% carrot. Trust me, they will love it. And you can experiment with more and more carrot, but take it slow. Once you push a kid too far or break them, it can be a hard road winning their confidence and trust back again.

Juices to flush the Liver, Gall Bladder and Kidneys: see Dr. Schulze's 5 Day Cleansing and Detoxification Program on pages 105-111.

3 CHAPTER THREE

VEGAN FOOD

The most powerful way to heal disease, detoxify and build your body is with Vegan Food. <u>Stop eating all Animals and Animal By-Products</u>.

WHY SHOULD I?

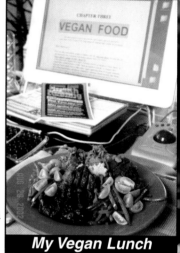

My Vegan Lunch

Over one and a half million people in America will die, **this year alone**, because the fat and cholesterol they consumed from eating animals KILLED THEM! **That is about 2 people EVERY MINUTE!**

It either physically clogged their heart's coronary arteries, giving them a heart attack, or clogged their cerebral arteries to their brain, giving them a stroke, or clogged other important blood supply lines to other major organs, depriving them of oxygen, nutrients and causing degeneration and disease. Cholesterol increases blood viscosity and blood platelet sticking (clotting), which kills by causing High Blood Pressure all the way to causing Cancer. Heart disease, stroke, most cancers, even prostate disease (BPH) and fibroid uterine tumors are now linked to eating animals. Most diseases are now found to be literally **"<u>diseases of the fork.</u>"** They're diseases caused by eating animals.

FACTS

- Over 10 Million Americans have now accepted the vegetarian food program and an additional 20 million are trying it out. Medical studies report that vegetarians are healthier, have less disease, need less doctor visits and less medication and <u>LIVE LONGER</u>! Do I need to go any further?

- The average American eats over: (12) three thousand pound cows, (6) whole pigs, (3,000) chickens, turkeys and other flying birds, (3,000) fish, sea creatures and sea scavengers and (30,000) quarts of cow's milk in their lifetime. Just imagine all of that dead decaying flesh and tissue going into your mouth, all of it passing through your digestive tract, into your bloodstream, your brain, your heart, and then out through your liver, bowel and kidneys.

- One average cubic inch of inspected choice beef has over 1,000 parasite larva in it, waiting to hatch inside your body.

- If you think that Chicken is a healthy alternative, every day in America 10 people die from food poisoning directly related to eating chicken and over an additional 10,000 get sick. Chicken is often billed as the healthy white meat alternative to red meat but this couldn't be a bigger lie. White meat chicken, even without the skin, ounce for ounce has just as much cholesterol as full fat hamburger meat. <u>Chicken also causes more food poisoning than any other type of meat consumed</u>.

- If you think that Fish is a healthy alternative, well, according to ABC's Prime Time Live report, two-thirds of all fresh fish tested, bought at various markets, was technically rotten. It had toxic levels of bacteria and parasites, even though it looked, smelled, and tasted normal. Another two-thirds tested positive for toxic levels of PCB's * (see below). 25% had toxic levels of mercury. They called Sushi a dangerous food.

- The University of Connecticut School of Medicine report blamed fish as the culprit in malignant breast cancer. They discovered that women with this malignancy had over double the concentrations of PCB's in their bodies. They warned against the intake of Fish and Dairy products and even added caution regarding the intake of ANY animal fat.

HOW TO DO IT?

Look, this is not about some moral crusade, animal rights, People for the Ethical Treatment of Animals, Greenpeace or Humane Society issue here. It's a simple life or death issue. Statistically, animal food is killing you more than anything else. It's a numbers game, and my job in the clinic is the same as writing this book for you, **to**

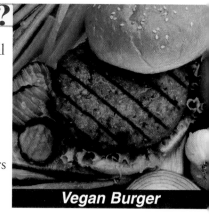

Vegan Burger

keep you alive. One of the best things I could do for them and now for you is to tell you to stop doing what the #1 contributing factor is to the #1 and #2 causes of death. In plain English, <u>stop eating what is killing you</u>.

Go ahead, add up all the causes of death—all the airplane crashes, auto accidents, poisoning, drowning, suicides, electrocution, drug overdoses, sky diving, street drugs, violent crime, AIDS, cancer—add up every other disease, all other causes of death and amazingly, *it doesn't even come close* to how many people die each year from heart attacks and stroke. It's numero uno and odds are it's going to kill you too.

Most oncologists feel that eating animals has caused our sky-rocketing rate of cancer, and you can add all the benign prostate growth (BPH) in men and uterine fibroid tumors in women, and a thousand other diseases, from diabetes to neuromuscular disorders, from Alzheimer's to arthritis. Clogging up your blood vessels. Clogging up your circulatory system. The vital system that delivers oxygen and nutrition—delivers life to your entire body—is all gummed up, all mucked up, all clogged up—from eating animals, from animal milk, eggs and by-products. And this is killing you, SO STOP IT.

If this seems a bit extreme, no, a heart attack caused by clogged arteries, that's extreme. No, a brain tumor caused by the growth hormones in steroids in the animal food you eat, that's extreme, because they're going to saw or drill the top of your head out to carve out that tumor. **Now that's extreme!** If this seems a bit final, you know, death is much more final. I want you to stop eating animals and their fluids and eggs. This is what I asked every one of my patients to do for three months when they began to work with me. Sure, I know that nobody ever died from eating one cheeseburger. But I am talking about a program here that will <u>heal disease</u> and <u>create powerful health</u> and **animal foods have no place on a healing or health program.** And any doctor that says otherwise is just afraid of pissing you off or making you uncomfortable or losing you as a patient because, believe me, the clinical and scientific proof is in, meat is dead.

Once my patients were healed, they could do and eat anything that they wanted. Some would go out and have a big steak. I never had to say a word, the steak did the talking and convincing for me. They felt so horrible after feeling so good, most of my patients then became vegetarians for life.

But regardless if you hate animals or are even a cattle rancher, just give me three months and I guarantee you will notice an amazing difference in how you feel.

THE VEGETARIAN FOOD PROGRAM

I have been a vegan for over 30 years. Stopping eating animal food literally saved my life and the lives of many of my patients. I use a vegan food program as a foundation to help people heal their diseases, regain their health and stay healthy. I use three different variations of a vegan food program.

#1 MY HEALTH BUILDING FOOD PROGRAM

#2 MY PURIFYING OR RAW FOOD PROGRAM

#3 JUICE FLUSHING OR JUICE FASTING

All three of these food programs are vegan vegetarian. My Health Building Food program is the best place for everyone to start, unless you are in immediate danger of dying. Then you would follow either my Purifying or Raw Food Program or more likely my Juice Flushing or Juice Fasting Program, both of which are described in Chapter Six, Cleansing and Detoxification.

THE HEALTH BUILDING FOOD PROGRAM

As I mentioned previously, all 3 food programs that I use are Vegan. That means they are totally vegetarian with no meat, fish, fowl, eggs or dairy products. To be very specific I mean no cows, pigs, lamb, horses, deer, elk, bear, turkey, chicken, duck, game birds, fish, clams, mussels, lobster, abalone, oysters, shrimp, scallops, calamari, sushi, chicken eggs, cow's milk, goat's milk, any animals parts, animal milks or animals fluids of any kind. I don't mean to insult your intelligence or be redundant but you would be as surprised as I was to see how many people thought that I certainly didn't mean lobster, or "aren't oysters supposed to be healthy" or "surely you didn't mean goat's milk, or yoghurt or kefir, aren't they health foods"? I even had one patient from Kazakhstan in the southern part of the old USSR who was drinking curdled horse milk for the first month and a half on his program with me until I discovered it. He said "well, it wasn't on your list of don'ts", and he was right. So after that experience I actually had an entire 8 1/2 by 11 sheet of paper for each patient that listed by name every type of animal food that existed and all animal byproducts known from sheep's brains and steak tartar, to haggis and braun for the Scotsmen. I would still add a new animal food every month or so when I discovered a new one. So the bottom line is that I cannot be clear enough on this issue.

Note: Our body manufactures all the cholesterol we need. It's when we eat extra cholesterol we hurt ourselves. The only source of dietary cholesterol is animal fat. **There is absolutely no cholesterol in any plant food.**

Another Note: Much of the pollution in the ground water and even air in the United States today can be directly related to the production of animal food and the agri-business that has to support it.

I know up to now I have talked a lot about the disease and death caused by eating animals. But eating a food program of Grains, Vegetables, Fruits, Beans, Legumes, Seeds, Nuts and Sprouts has an equal and opposite *upside*. A healthy food program is the foundation of Natural Healing. Notice I didn't say *a* foundation, I said *the* foundation.

Eating this type of food gives you maximum nutrition with the minimum digestive effort without any toxic pollution of your body. There are also many other attributes to this vegetarian food program, like fiber. Fiber has many healing benefits including helping your entire digestive tract work better, especially your bowel elimination. Absolutely NO animal food contains ANY Fiber; it only exists in the plant world.

My Health Building Food Program is my most lenient and varied food program. That is why it is the best one to start on. It is also the best maintenance food program, the one you will usually stay on about 48 weeks a year. This is because it is best to take a week out of every season and follow my Purifying Food Program and Juice Flushing. My patients who followed this type of food program regime maintained powerful health.

The only exception would be that if you get ill, you would immediately stop the Health Building Food Program and begin the Purifying Food Program. If you are really ill you would stop all solid food and move into my Juice Flushing Program.

**Again the Health Building Food Program is designed to supply your body with optimum nutrition in a manner which is easy to digest and assimilate. The food on this program is not toxic or congestive to your body in any way, but will not generally initiate a cleanse or detoxification either**.

The Health Building Food Program consists of all Grains, Vegetables, Fruits Beans, Legumes, Seeds, Nuts and Sprouts. They can be either Raw, Sprouted, Steamed or Cooked. At first to the novice this may not seem like a lot of food or food choices but you will see that there is an almost unlimited array of food choices and menu options on this program. Veggie chili soy cheeseburgers, spaghetti, and baked potatoes are totally legal on this program and as you begin to use your imagination you will find that this food program is totally sustainable and easily followed.

As you are working towards making this food program your new way of life it is important to be very receptive and positive about the new types of food that you may eat and be imaginative and inventive about the preparation of them. Most people don't eat a cold hamburger on a plate with nothing on it so remember to enjoy herbs and spices and all the many great sauces and condiments that are available in the health food store. Also remember to invent and make your own and, most importantly, keep your sense of humor.

Visit the health food store more like a museum and always leave yourself plenty of time to browse around. There are new products coming out every week and many of them are great, some are not so great, and some you might be better off steaming and eating the box and throwing out the contents, but in any case try everything! Enjoy yourself and make this a positive, exciting adventure into your new, healthy way of living. Everything sold in a health food store is not necessarily healthy, but it will always be better than its counterpart in a regular grocery store (less fat, salt, sugar, artificial colorings, flavorings and dangerous preservatives etc). Keep reading the product labels, even in the health food store.

Note: Remember, it's not what you do on holidays, New Years, Your Birthday or Saturday night that counts. It's what you do 6 days a week that decides your level of health.

THE HEALTH BUILDING MORNING

I always suggest to start each day with 8 to 16 ounces of pure water. This will flush your digestive tract of any leftover digestive juices and food. It is also the best way to lubricate and cleanse your body, and a great time to do it is when you are breaking the fast, breakfast.

Next I suggest some type of blender drink. To gulp down a piece of toast or eat some cereal first thing in the morning sets our digestive tract off to six hours of hard labor. This is why most people feel tired all morning and then need coffee to keep them going. Start your day off instead with a nutritional morning drink that assimilates fast, getting your blood packed with vitamins, minerals, enzymes, amino acids and hundreds of other nutrition substances that give you energy.

For 35 years now I have been playing around, making hundreds of different variations of my morning blender drink. Most people are not as obsessed as I am with nutrition, adding a little bit of this and that.

But in the clinic, making morning drinks for my patients was a very serious business. Many of my patients were anemic from Leukemia and other diseases. If they didn't get their nutrition, they could be dead by nightfall. I had a couple problems I had to overcome with these patients.

First, they were so sick that they had very little if any digestive ability. Their digestive ability was bad because of Liver Cancer, Pancreatic Cancer, Chronic Stomach Ulcers, and many had literally burned out digestive tracts from years on extremely harsh medical drugs.

Secondly, even if they could digest a vitamin pill, they didn't stand a chance at assimilating it. After all, it's not really how much you take of a particular nutrient that makes the difference; the question is how much of that nutrient you took actually got into your blood and bloodstream and got to the dying cells that need it. **In other words it's not how much you** *take*, **but how much you** *assimilate*.

So to keep these patients alive, many years ago in my clinic I did lots of experimentation with juicing, juicers, juices and juice combinations. Without a doubt, fresh organic juice kept my patients alive. I have said it many times, it is like a natural healing blood transfusion.

Regardless, some of my patients still died and others obviously needed something even more nutritionally concentrated and powerful than just juice. That is when I started investigating food supplements that were extremely high in particular vitamins and minerals. I was also looking at single cell foods like spirulina, chlorella, sachromyces cervisiae nutritional yeast and others that were not only super foods and that were the highest in particular nutrients, but also were *single-celled*, ones that could be assimilated into your blood, assimilated right in your mouth before they even reach your intestines. I knew immediately these foods and herbs were the missing answer that I needed for my sickest patients.

I eventually designed a food powder I simply called SuperFood that I had my sickest patients add to their morning juice in a last ditch desperate attempt to keep them alive. Well, it not only kept them alive, they thrived. So I started using it with all of my patients and within a year people were demanding and ordering it from all over the world. Today I sell my SuperFood along with many of my other herbal formulae through my company, the American Botanical Pharmacy. If it is not from this company, it is not mine, period.

Anyway, advertisement over, the following is a simple beginning morning drink formula you can start your Health Building Food Program with.

THE NUTRITIONAL MORNING DRINK

- **8 ounces of FRESH squeezed fruit juice**
- **8 ounces of distilled or purified water**
- **1/2 to 1 cup of fresh fruit (banana, papaya, apple, pear, berries etc.)**
- **2 level tablespoons of SUPERFOOD Organic Vitamin and Mineral Concentrate**

Blend it up for just a minute and drink slowly, swishing each mouthful. Now this is the real *breakfast of champions.*

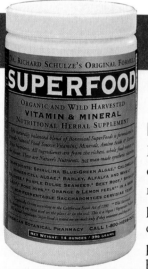

Dr. Schulze's
SUPERFOOD

100% Organic Vitamin & Mineral Food Concentrate

MODERN LIFE CAN BEAT YOU UP.

Most people today live on a diet of over-processed and over-cooked food, not to mention coffee, sugar, chocolate, junk food, prescription drugs and alcohol. Our environment is more toxic, has more chemical pollutants in it and less oxygen than ever before. Most of us suffer from lack of exercise, lack of sleep and unheard of levels of stress. This constant bombardment we call modern living devours nutrients like a raging forest fire with a 100 m.p.h. tailwind.

EVERY PATIENT THAT WALKED INTO MY CLINIC WAS NUTRITIONALLY DEPLETED.

A lack of nutrition in your blood can cause everything from low energy and a weak immune system to virtually any disease. Your speed and ability to recover are greatly reduced when you are nutritionally depleted. Nutrition is what builds every cell, every organ and every metabolic chemical in your body. Nutrition is what builds your body; it's what YOU are made of. Having a rich supply of nutrition in your blood gives you energy, vitality, strength, protects you from disease and illness, and if you get sick, speeds up your recovery dramatically.

IT'S NOT HOW MUCH YOU TAKE, BUT HOW MUCH YOU ASSIMILATE.

Even in perfect health it is difficult to digest and assimilate vitamin and mineral pills, but if you're sick, you don't stand a chance. So in the clinic it didn't take long for me to discover that vitamin and mineral pills were NOT helping any of my patients get well. They were literally throwing their money down the toilet.

We are currently entering a new era of nutrition. It is no longer a matter of how many milligrams you take of this or that nutrient, but how much of what you are taking is actually ending up in your bloodstream and getting to the organs that need it.

I designed and developed SUPERFOOD using numerous single-celled microplants. What this means in plain English is that you can assimilate it in minutes, right into your blood, where you need it. Again, it's not how much you take in milligrams or international units of a particular nutrient that's important, but how much of that nutrient you swallow gets into your bloodstream and to your cells where you need it.

QUESTIONS AND FEARS ABOUT BECOMING A VEGETARIAN

Many of my patients were professional athletes, dancers, body builders, yoga teachers and students. Almost daily I was asked the same questions regarding being a vegetarian:

Is there enough PROTEIN in a vegetarian diet?

Will I have enough ENERGY?

Where will I get my CALCIUM without drinking milk or using dairy products?

PROTEIN: In regards to necessary protein consumption, a vegetarian diet has an overabundance. This brings up three very interesting protein facts:

#1 Any food program or diet that has sufficient caloric intake to sustain life also has a sufficient protein amount. In fact, it is impossible to create a food program that has enough calories but is deficient in protein.

#2 High protein was a misguided nutritional fad of the 1950's. Many erroneously believed that a healthy person should consume 75 to 100 grams of protein a day. Today it is highly agreed on that all of this protein actually created many diseases and made many people sick and today a low protein diet is known to be the safest, healthiest and the most promotive of longevity.

Interestingly, most of this supposedly scientific but very wrong high protein *dietary advice* has now been traced back to the overzealous promoters at the beef and dairy industries. A similar example is that in the 1930's cigarettes were proclaimed by medical doctors to soothe throat inflammation and white refined sugar was proclaimed an official food group, again, by medical doctors. I wonder who was paying them to lie?

#3 In a book by Frances Moore Lappe the protein issue was again misguided. In this book the author stated that you must eat complete proteins and, if you don't, then you must combine proteins in the same meal (like beans and rice) that add up to all of the 8 essential amino acids making up a complete protein. This is simply hogwash. It has been scientifically disproved and even the author has retracted this bad theory years later, but I still hear people every day spouting this nonsense.

In the last 20 years, teams of medical researchers from Harvard, The American Dietetic Association, The American Medical Association and most other major conservative medical groups have studied the vegetarian diet. All of them came to the same conclusion, that the vegetarian diet was "well above sufficient" in protein and all other essential nutrients, even for pregnant women and growing children and teenagers.

So I hope we can put this protein issue to rest, forever!

ENERGY: As far as the energy vs. protein intake issue, it seems to be a psychological issue, not a physiological one. In other words it seems to be all in people's minds.

It appears that all the brainwashing by the Beef Advisory Board and the American Dairy Council has paid off again, as with the protein issue. <u>Many people seem to feel that protein gives us quick energy, but there is no scientific data or evidence to substantiate this feeling</u>. Vegetable protein is essential for growth, repair and building new tissue, but it is complex carbohydrates, starch and sugars that give us energy. This is why carbohydrate loading is practiced by many professional athletes, especially marathon runners. This is using a very high carbohydrate diet in the days before athletic competition or extensive workouts. It is mainly complex carbohydrates, especially grains and vegetables, that your body converts to glycogen and stores for future energy needs. When needed, your body converts this glycogen to the sugar glucose which is needed for muscular work, muscular contraction and energy.

In my clinic I heard many people say that they used to be vegetarians but they had to go back and start eating meat again because they needed *more protein* or *more energy*. Since there is absolutely no scientific or medical basis for this phenomenon, and after ~~interrogating~~, I mean interviewing, these patients, I always discovered that it was simply because the patient just wanted to eat meat again.

It may have been a comfort food for them or just a family tradition but in this day and age it is not cool anymore to say "I started eating veal again because my family is Italian and it makes me feel warm and fuzzy all over." It is much more politically correct but *medically incorrect* to just say, "I didn't have enough energy, I needed more protein." Or the newest bull, I'm an O Blood type, I am supposed to eat meat.

CALCIUM: And finally, the calcium issue. Calcium is needed by the body to build strong bones and teeth and to assist in numerous other extremely important metabolic functions. Our bones are comprised of about 85% calcium. Bone deterioration and brittleness seems to be caused by two major factors, not enough easy-to-assimilate calcium in our diets (like vegetables instead of oyster shells and ground up rocks) and back to protein, too much protein intake.

I am not going to write an in-depth metabolic essay here on how protein intake negatively affects your calcium uptake, but let me just tell you the basics.

When you consume a food that contains calcium your body digests it and the calcium enters into your blood. After an amount of time, if there is excess calcium in your blood that you don't need, it is taken out of your blood and deposited into your bones. Your bones and skeletal system not only structurally support your body, but they also serve as a calcium depository and calcium storage reserve.

The metabolic downside of consuming too much protein is that to metabolize this protein your kidneys remove your blood calcium and you urinate it away and it doesn't get a chance to be deposited into your bones. This is simply why meat eaters have double the bone loss and osteoporosis than vegetarians.

While misinformed doctors and animal industry advertisements tell women to ingest MORE calcium and animal food to treat and prevent osteoporosis, the real metabolic solution is to simply consume LESS protein. This is why milk is NOT a good choice as a calcium supplement, because it is also high in protein, the calcium in milk doesn't end up getting to your bones.

Carrot juice and Orange juice have almost the identical calcium content as milk, ounce for ounce, but their much lower protein content makes them excellent calcium supplements. They can be assimilated better because they have a low protein content and have none of the negative side effects from lactose intolerance to mucous promotion. Many grains, vegetables and fruits are rich sources of calcium also.

After a career of promoting cow's milk to mothers for their children (because in the 1950's breast feeding was at the top of the politically INcorrect list in America), the very famous medical doctor and pediatrician Dr. Benjamin Spock finally reversed his decision before he died and said that not only does he not suggest giving newborns, or any children, cow's milk, but he even went as far as to say that he didn't feel it was a good source of calcium because he felt it was hard to digest and that he felt it wasn't a good food.

Hard mineral calcium supplements are also very difficult to impossible for your body to assimilate. I see many people using calcium supplements like oyster shell and other similar substances that are 99% inassimilable.

LIVE FOOD HIGH IN CALCIUM

Kale	Seaweed
Broccoli	Collard greens
Spinach	Turnip greens
Sesame seeds	Mustard greens
Kelp	White beans

A final interesting note is that in most medical studies vegetarians have much stronger bones. **Reports on studies from The Medical Tribune and The Journal of Clinical Nutrition show conclusively that by age 65, meat eaters have over double the bone loss and deterioration than vegetarians.** This is partly due to the higher protein intake of meat eaters.

FACT

- The United States Department of Agriculture states that the average American vegetarian consumes 150% of their needed protein requirements and the average meat eater consumes 200%, or twice what they need. Studies show that this increase in protein consumption, even milk, CAUSES osteoporosis, not cures it.

4 CHAPTER FOUR

LIVE FOOD

Eat more raw food

WHY SHOULD I?

Live food equals life. It is filled with enzymes, vitamins, and hundreds of other nutritional substances that are destroyed by heating, cooking and the processing of food. Eating food raw and sprouted gives you a nutritional blast that is second only to juices.

Eating live food brings life back into your body.

FACTS

- Enzymes are life-giving nutrients in all foods. Heating food and Cooking food destroys all the enzymes.

- Most Vitamins are totally destroyed or at least severely depleted by heating and cooking.

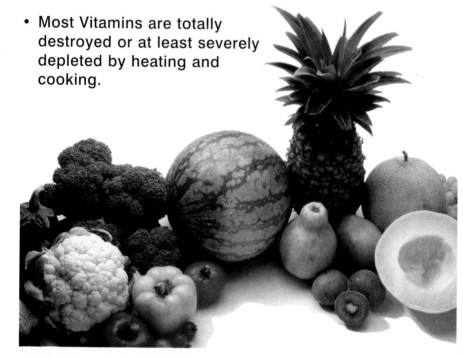

How To Do It?

FIRST A STORY FROM MY GARDEN

Since my son Arthur is home schooled, every year as part of our learning we grow food. I have about an acre that I devote to our organic garden project. We have about 100 fruit trees growing on the terraced hill, Avocado, Orange, Lemon, Lime, Sweet Lime, Grapefruit, Tangerine, Kumquats, Figs, Plums, Nectarines, Peaches, Apricots, Persimmons, Pomegranites, Cheramoyas, Loquats, Apples, Pears, Olives and even Macadamia nuts. On the flat land we grow Corn, Watermelon, Squash, Potatoes, Tomatoes, Hot Peppers and many other vegetables. We also grow organic herbs to subsidize what American Botanical Pharmacy needs, like Echinacea, Fennel, Rosemary, Lavender, Tea Tree, and others. My first point is that anyone, with a little help from the kids, can grow enough food for the whole neighborhood. Let's not let growing food become a lost art or we will all be in a lot of trouble.

For my son it is an illuminating experience, composting and recycling, preparing and feeding the earth, and the fun part, irrigation. A few years ago he planted a small sunflower seed only to grow a 10 foot high massive plant with a stalk as big around as his arm. Looking up at this huge sunflower he asked me *"how could one little seed make this huge plant?"* That's a very good question. Well, one big reason is God and Nature, and also enzymes inside the seed. He looked at me and said, **"Wow, there must be a lot of LIFE inside that seed."** I couldn't have said it better myself.

One of my great teachers, the late Dr. Bernard Jensen, among many others, used to always promote when eating grapes, apples, watermelons or almost any food to also chew and eat the seeds. This great doctor knew that the seeds contained the life. Isn't it interesting that today, many of the fruits are being grown seedless, for eating convenience, obviously not nutrition.

WHY EAT RAW FOOD

Life Energy, Life Force, Enzymes, whatever you want to call it, is something that we seemed to have forgotten. Go ahead, dig a hole, plant a vitamin, or a mineral, or a hamburger, or a loaf of bread, or any cooked food for that matter, and what happens? Nothing! You can water it, feed it, chant or even sleep over it and absolutely nothing is going to happen, except that it is going to rot. But plant a little sunflower seed and look out, a massive explosion of life is about to happen, you are going to get something twice as tall as you! Plant a raw almond and you will get a huge tree!

For this reason alone eating live, raw food, food that is filled with this Life Force, Life Energy, Enzymes and Plant Phytochemicals that create growth and life, nourishes your body in a much more powerful way than any cooked food.

Some boring scientist might laugh and say that this is just genetics, but what feeds the genetics? These are the same scientists that think they are so smart and have come so far but I have yet to see just one of them be able to synthesize even a pea in the laboratory. They might come up with some brown goo that they claim has the same exact elements and nutrients as a pea, but what will happen if you plant it? You won't get more peas, SOMETHING IS MISSING, and that missing factor is Life Energy, Life Force, Enzymes, God, Nature, Phytochemicals or whatever other name you want to put on it.

So what's my point? LIVE FOOD CREATES LIFE, so **EAT MORE LIVE, RAW FOODS.**

If the last step, Step #3, being a vegetarian, was a big leap for you, then don't push yourself too hard into eating raw foods too fast. A great way to ensure your success on any program, especially the ones that I suggest in this book that are for life, is to make slow, wide, easy and big turns. If you turn on a dime like going from a full-fledged carnivore to a fruitarian overnight, chances are you will be putting bacon in your morning drink tomorrow. You changed too fast. Come on, you should know your ability to change by now and what's real and what won't last. Don't bullshit yourself.

So if this type of food program is very different, alien and all new to you, just be a vegetarian for now like I discussed in the last chapter.

I don't care if you hardly eat any raw or live food at all right now. Just having your morning SuperFood drink gives you plenty of live, raw, enzyme-rich food and nutrition, so take it easy. Eat anything you want, as long as it's vegetarian.

As you feel more comfortable with not eating meat, I want you to add more live and raw food into your life. As you stabilize, add more live food. As you feel better about your food program, eat more live food.

Start adding a side of grated raw beets, or raw carrots, or raw cabbage, or all three, to your cooked vegetarian lunch. Please add some herbs, garlic, raw organic unfiltered apple cider vinegar and some extra-virgin, cold-first-pressing olive oil. It will make everything taste better. Soon you'll be adding so much life and live food into your body you won't believe the amount of energy you have. Just by having your morning drink every day that I described in the last chapter and by adding some live food to your lunch and dinner, your health level, your world, is going to change by what you are not putting into your mouth and what you are beginning to eat.

Besides eating raw fruits and vegetables, you can soak and sprout any Grains, Beans, Legumes, Seeds or Nuts. This makes them more digestible and starts the enzyme action. If you need more inspiration and recipes there are many raw food uncook books available. A few of my favorites are:

1. John Robbins, for information, not necessarily recipes.
2. Light Eating for Survival, by Maria Acciardo. An old book but I love it. I used to give it to every one of my patients. Good, simple recipes.

A DR. JOHN R. CHRISTOPHER SHORT STORY

Many, many years ago, when Dr. John Christopher was still alive, he was coming to Los Angeles to speak at a very large nutritional convention. In his day he was one of a few health speakers, like Dr. Bernard Jensen, that would literally draw thousands and thousands of people. Sure he had great teachers and a good education in his respective field, but his ability to draw huge crowds was simply because he had helped thousands and thousands of people all over America heal their diseases using Natural Healing and Herbal Medicine. He *was the man!* Often hundreds of people would literally panic, fight and even climb over each other to get close to him. It got rough a few times so I was not only his apprentice and the senior teacher at his School of Natural Healing in Utah, but because of my extensive background in the Martial Arts, I was also his bodyguard on occasion.

Since I lived near Los Angeles I was to pick him and his son up at the airport and take him to this Nutritional convention where he was the guest of honor and main speaker. Most conventions he spoke at were Health Conventions, not *nutritional product conventions,* but like me, he would go almost anywhere people who wanted to hear his healing message asked him to go.

We arrived at the convention a few hours early so he wanted to walk around and look at all of the booths that were representing the biggest nutritional companies of the era and also selling their products. Booths filled with Vitamins, Minerals, Enzymes, Amino Acids, all in pill and powder form with the brightest and most polished looking labels and sharp, well-dressed sales people. Obviously the main reason for having a convention of this sort is to exhibit your nutritional products for the industry, the health food store owners and the consumer, *the buyers.* And of course take orders and sell them.

The time came for Dr. Christopher to speak, the very large convention room was already overcrowded and many people were now a bit frantic that he was on stage and that they didn't have a seat so they were pushing and shoving themselves in every doorway.

Dr. Christopher, in his usual three piece *wool* suit, (in the time when polyester was king), white shirt, tie, gold watch chain and highly polished shoes, was introduced and walked a few steps to the podium. The crowd leapt to their feet and erupted in deafening screams, cheers and applause. He cleared his throat and said *(since it was about 25 years ago and a very intense moment I am telling you what he said to the best of my memory),* "Good afternoon, and thank you for asking me to speak here today" (he was always a very polite man). Within what felt like a minute, if that, he said, *"as I have been walking around this wonderful and very large convention hall today I have met some very nice people. I have also seen many different products but the only problem is that*

everything I have seen at every booth and on every table . . . . IS DEAD!"
As he yelled DEAD he hit the podium with his fist and the microphone
fed back and the sound of his fist hitting the wood reverberated
throughout this huge room.

Holy live food shit, Batman! I was shocked, as were the thousands and
thousands of people in the room, and within what seemed like two
seconds you could have heard a pin drop in this huge room. It was <u>dead
silent</u>. I moved very quickly towards the podium like a secret service
agent would to block a bullet being fired at the President. The people in
the room were starting to grumble and as I remember it the great old
Dr. Christopher was not phased and started to continue his *illuminating*
lecture. At that moment I believe someone on stage jumped in and said
the thank you very much, hook around the neck, quick, change the
subject fast, start saying something else, and others shuttled the doc off
the stage.

I thought that he had made a mistake and forgot where he was or
pulled out the wrong speaking notes for the next city and the next
convention, but he knew exactly where he was, exactly what he was
doing and exactly what he was saying. Later that afternoon he said
something to me like, *"Well, someone had to tell them so I figured it might
as well be me"*.

Since that day I have been barred from speaking at this particular
nutritional convention and many others just by my association with the
great Dr. Christopher, and I am very proud of this guilt by association.

GARLIC

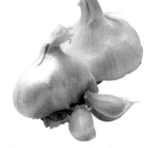

In the clinic and with my own
healing I have learned that Garlic is truly
a miracle plant. If I were to be restricted
to only a handful of herbs, Garlic,
Cayenne, Lobelia and Aloe would be on
the top of the list, <u>in that order</u>!

For powerful health start adding raw Garlic into your food program.
Take it easy at first and finely chop up little pieces and sneak them into
your food. In no time you will probably become a Garlic junky like

myself and start eating large amounts of it. When I cook, actually heat food and cook, I will add 4 to 6 BULBS or about 100 cloves of garlic to a curry or a pasta sauce that I am making, for 3 or 4 people. When cooking with Garlic, don't be a wimp. Heat *destroys* a lot of Garlic's taste, intensity and medicinal action so always use a lot if you are going to cook it. When visiting Los Angeles or San Francisco, try eating at the Stinking Rose Restaurant to see some of the possibilities of Garlic Cuisine.

But since it is my favorite healing herb and also one of my favorite foods I would like to tell you a little more about it's medicinal power. This may encourage you to add more of this wonderful, miraculous and healing plant in your life.

A great healing dose is at least 3 cloves of FRESH, RAW Garlic every day.

Garlic, known botanically as Allium sativum, is certainly one of nature's miracle plants. It has been worshiped since the beginning of recorded history for its ability to heal and strengthen the body. The ancient Egyptians, Greeks and Romans all used garlic in copious amounts to increase strength and combat disease and illness. Hippocrates, the so-called father of modern medicine, was actually an herbalist and natural healer. He used garlic specifically to treat cancer. As recently as World War I and II, when sulphur drugs were used on battle wounds, when there was a shortage, the British government used garlic in the battlefield hospitals. It is credited with saving thousands of lives. It was used in various preparations to disinfect and heal battle wounds and also used internally to successfully treat typhoid fever and dysentery.

Today garlic is the leading over the counter drug in many European and Asian countries. It is an official drug in many countries and prescribed by medical doctors outside the U.S. for many diseases, especially hypertension (high blood pressure), high cholesterol, cancer, and, especially, as a broad spectrum anti-biotic, anti-viral agent and fungicide. It was eliminated from medical use during the last century in the United States, not because of its inability to heal, but due to pressure on doctors from the AMA and the pharmaceutical companies. For years the pharmaceutical industry and the American Medical Association have been attempting to discourage the public from using plants to heal themselves, in fact discouraging any home or self-treating of disease to make you more doctor and drug-dependent. It seems that even the tight fist from these two groups and the trillion dollars a year they demand can't keep garlic underground anymore.

GARLIC AND HEART DISEASE

Garlic is famous for it's healing power with heart disease. Heart disease is the #1 cause of death in the United States today. This year almost 1 million people will die from it. That's about 2 people a minute. 99% of all these heart deaths are caused by cholesterol and saturated fat blocking the coronary arteries. Attention was first put on garlic as a cardiac remedy when researchers noticed that in countries that had high garlic consumption, ***the incidence of heart disease was much lower than average.***

Garlic has been found to lower serum cholesterol and triglyceride levels and reduce the build-up of atherosclerotic plaque in our arteries. It does this partly by increasing our blood levels of high density lipo-proteins (HDL's). These lipo-proteins clear our blood of excess cholesterol and fat. Garlic also lowers our low density lipo-proteins (LDL's), which can attribute to arterial plaque.

Medical researchers have also found substances in garlic that inhibit blood platelet aggregation (the sticking together of blood cells). This is just another way that garlic can reduce your risk of heart attack.

High blood pressure is a worldwide epidemic and in every study garlic has proven conclusively to reduce hypertension. Because of its powerful effect on blood pressure, the Japanese Food and Drug Administration has approved garlic and it is now an official drug listed in the Japanese Pharmacopeia.

If you are looking for a safe and effective remedy for heart disease, Garlic is a great choice. Whether you have high blood pressure, high cholesterol and triglycerides, arterial plaque or clotting, Garlic is for you.

GARLIC AND CANCER

Garlic has proven to be an effective cancer therapy. One-third of all the medical research into garlic is cancer-related. The National Cancer Institute has reported that cancer incidence worldwide is lowest in the countries where garlic consumption is the highest: France, Spain and Italy. In the few isolated rural areas of the world where there is NO incidence of cancer, the garlic consumption was also the highest reported.

Garlic has been shown to help our white blood cells not only defend us against cancer, but also to increase our ability to destroy tumors.

When the powerful healing phytochemicals of garlic are present in the bloodstream, many aspects of our immunity are enhanced. Garlic not only destroys bacteria, virus and fungus on contact but it also stimulates cellular immunity. This is why I chose it as a compliment to Echinacea in my **Echinacea Plus Tonic Formula**. Garlic has proven in the laboratory to stimulate the production of interferon, a natural immune chemical that has been used in cancer treatment and also enhance natural killer cells that destroy cancer and tumors. Therefore Garlic inhibits and stops tumor growth, and even reduces the associated pain of cancer.

Colon-rectal cancer is on the rise. In many areas of the world it is the #1 cancer among men and women together as a group. According to The Merck Manual almost 1/2 of all American adults over age 50 have diverticulosis (bowel herniation). **Garlic has been found in double blind studies to reduce the incidence of colon-rectal cancer.** Garlic has also been reported to reduce stomach cancer. **In one medical university study garlic was shown to reduce stomach cancer 10 times more effectively than the non-garlic eating group.**

Garlic, with its over 80 different sulphur compounds, is a free radical scavenger. This is just another way that garlic will protect you from cancer and suppress chemically-induced cancers.

GARLIC AND DISEASE CAUSING MICRO-ORGANISMS

Garlic is a powerful Antibiotic, Anti-Viral and Anti-Fungal agent.

Garlic is a very powerful anti-biotic. Garlic juice diluted 1 part in 125,000 has been found to inhibit the growth of bacteria. Garlic destroys BOTH gram-positive and gram-negative bacteria, making it a broad spectrum antibiotic. Garlic's successful long term use as an anti-bacterial agent in Russia has awarded it the nickname of Russian penicillin.

Pharmaceutical antibiotics are non-selective in their destruction of bacteria in your body; they just destroy it all. This creates many problems because our body has many so-called *friendly* bacteria that we need for proper metabolic functions. This is why many people, after a course of antibiotic therapy, have digestive problems, constipation, and yeast and fungal overgrowth infections. Our bodies also become immune to these antibiotics over time and sometimes dangerous resistant strains of bacteria are actually created in our body.

Garlic is totally selective in its bacteria destruction, only killing bacteria that's harmful to our body. What is amazing is that at the same time garlic actually enhances our friendly bacteria and improves our intestinal flora and digestion.

Garlic destroys many types of bacteria including Streptococcus, Staphylococcus, Typhoid, Diphtheria, Cholera, Bacterial Dysentery (Traveler's diarrhea), Tuberculosis, Tetanus, Rheumatic bacteria, and many others.

Some say that the reason you don't catch colds when you eat garlic is because no one will come near you. Regardless, **Garlic is also a powerful anti-viral agent.** Many feel it's the cure for the common cold because it destroys various viruses that cause upper respiratory infections and influenza.

Garlic destroys, on contact, the viral infections of Measles, Mumps, Mononucleosis, Chicken pox, Herpes simplex #1 and #2, Herpes zoster, Viral Hepatitis, Scarlet fever, Rabies and others.

Garlic's anti-fungal ability is second to none. In the laboratory it has proved to be more potent than any known anti-fungal agent, including Nystatin. Garlic will regulate the overgrowth of Candida albicans.

5 CHAPTER FIVE

BOWEL CLEANSING

You should have one bowel movement per day for every meal you eat.

WHY SHOULD I?

From your mouth to your anus, your intestines are as long as two cars parked end to end. Since Americans have the highest incidence of colon disease and cancer in the world, <u>knowing what goes on in the last 5 feet of your intestines can</u> **SAVE YOUR LIFE!**

FACTS

- COLON CANCER **KILLS 400%** more people than **AIDS.** It actually KILLS more men and women in America than breast cancer or prostate cancer.

THE AVERAGE AMERICAN'S COLON

COLITIS

many DIVERTICULI

DIVERTICULITIS (inflamed and leaking DIVERTICULI)

STRICTURE

POLYPS

PROLAPSED TRANSVERSE COLON

SPASTIC DESCENDING COLON

CANCER

HERNIATED CECUM (caused by constipation; favorite home for parasites)

HERNIATED SIGMOID (from constipation)

APPENDIX IMPACTION (with fecal matter, causing appendicitis)

BLEEDING RECTAL FISSURES

HEMORRHOIDS

- **100%** of **Americans** eventually have **DIVERTICULOSIS** or many **DIVERTICULI.**

- Up to **50%** of **Americans** have **POLYPS** in their **COLON.**

- COLON RECTAL CANCER will **KILL** about **60,000 Americans** this year with over **130,000** new cases diagnosed.

- In my clinic **80%** of my patients' diseases were gone after they did my **BOWEL DETOXIFICATION PROGRAM.**

HOW TO DO IT?

Let's check what the
TOP MEDICAL DOCTORS SAY...

The Merck Manual is written by the most distinguished and respected group of medical doctors in the world and published by one of the largest pharmaceutical manufacturers in the world. It is the medical industry's standard text for the diagnosis and treatment of disease. **This book tells us that colon degeneration is on the rise**.

The incidence of diverticulosis (herniated bowel pockets caused by constipation) has increased dramatically over the past 50 years. It states that in 1950 only 10% of adults over the age of 45 had this disease; in 1955, 15%; in 1972, 30%; and in 1987, 45%. The most recent edition states that the incidence increases rapidly over age 40 and that **every person will have diverticulosis if they live long enough**.

EVERY AMERICAN eventually has DIVERTICULOSIS or has many DIVERTICULA

Diverticuli are sac-like herniations through the muscular wall of the colon that are caused by increased pressure in the bowel from constipation. By old age every American has many. **They are filled with trapped fecal sludge, they become infected, and the rotting feces erodes the surrounding mucousa. Blood vessels rupture, then infection begins**.

UP TO 50% OF AMERICANS have POLYPS in their COLON

A Polyp is a tumor that arises from the bowel surface and protrudes into the inside of the colon. **Most polyps eventually transform into malignant cancer tumors**.

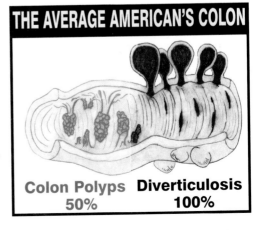

THE AVERAGE AMERICAN'S COLON

Colon Polyps 50%   Diverticulosis 100%

"HOW BAD CAN IT GET?
MY CONSTIPATION RECORD BREAKERS."

Thirty years ago when I first heard the great Dr. Christopher speak about extreme constipation, I thought he was lying. I wanted to believe him, but when he told me that he had patients that hadn't had a bowel movement in a month, well, I thought that he was telling me a natural healing fish story.

But, in the first year of running my Hollywood clinic, I had a fashion model come to see me, a very beautiful girl, slim, 5'8" and 115 pounds, and she only had **1 BOWEL MOVEMENT A MONTH** for the past year and a half. I was shocked! Where did it go? I was ready to call David Copperfield or Sigfried and Roy. This was real magic.

That year I had many patients that only had 1 bowel movement a month, and for a few years in the clinic that was the record, until a woman came to see me, a 38 year-old attorney that only went every other month. She had **ONLY 6 BOWEL MOVEMENTS IN A YEAR!** She held the record for a while, but then there was a young woman from Santa Rosa, California. She only had 3 bowel movements during her last pregnancy. That's one bowel movement per trimester and

only two others that year. Now the record holder was **ONLY 5 BOWEL MOVEMENTS IN A YEAR.** That held the record for some time, but three years ago I got a letter from a lady in Southern California thanking me for my Intestinal Formula #1. In the letter, she stated that before using my herbal formula she was only having one bowel movement every 6 months. **THAT IS ONLY 2 BOWEL MOVEMENTS A YEAR, THE CURRENT RECORD HOLDER!!!!!**

Sure, the above were extreme cases, but most of my patients suffered from some sort of constipation. I had well over a thousand patients that were lucky if they went once a week. People who are constipated live in discomfort, fear and shame. They usually don't go around talking about it and don't know where to turn. Everyone has failed them: the empty promises of their medical doctors, their toxic mineral oil, the wimpy herbal laxatives that couldn't even make you fart, and the natural healers with their bran. Give me a break! They pay the money, and could fill a bus with the bottles of drugs and herbs that they took, **BUT THEY STILL COULDN'T POOP UNTIL THEY MET ME.**

The average American stores from six to ten pounds of fecal waste in their colon, which is not healthy. As far as the record breaking accumulation of fecal matter, I had one man in Hawaii who got his dosage up to 46 capsules of my now famous Intestinal Formula #1, which is a record in itself, before his bowels moved. Then that night, sitting on the toilet, HE EVACUATED 56 POUNDS OF FECAL MATTER. I met his wife and she said to me that she always knew her husband was full of shit (her words, not mine), but was she right. I had one lady who, after a year of my herbal bowel cleansing program, lost over 200 pounds. She went from 410 pounds down to 180.

A 5 FOOT LONG FECAL IMPACTION REMOVED WITH DR. SCHULZE'S INTESTINAL DETOXIFICATION PROGRAM

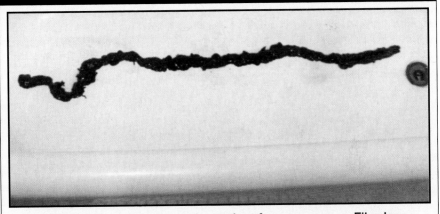

This impaction had been in the patient for many years. Fiberless food sludge that is mostly animal food and refined flour enters your colon. Because of constipation and infrequent bowel movements, it is not completely eliminated. The remainder of it plasters onto the inside wall of your colon. That is why in this picture the fecal casing took on the shape of the inside of this patient's bowel including the colon's folds and herniated diverticula.

This process can literally go on for decades just like an old steel water pipe that gathers corrosion over years and its inside diameter shrinks. Constipation is a progressively degenerating disease where eventually, you have total blockage of the colon or colon disease, often causing cancer and death. I have seen this type of fecal mucoid casing come out of many of the chronically constipated patients in my clinic, but usually not after their first Intestinal Detoxification Program. Often like with this man, it took 4 or 5 times. This man is fine and healthy now, and his lower abdomen that was distended for years is now flat. I estimate that this was 10 to 15 years of backed up fecal sludge.

"WHAT THE HECK IS A NORMAL POOP ANYWAY?"

NORMAL FREQUENCY

I have literally traveled around the world in search of what a normal bowel movement and bowel habit should be like. Now, how many people can say that? I have traveled from the remote jungles of Central America to India, China, almost everywhere to discover what is normal because I knew I wasn't going to find normal in New York, California and not even in Iowa. I wanted to see primitive people living in rural, non-industrialized areas, living simple natural rural lives under very little stress, getting moderate amounts of exercise and eating simple natural diets of locally foraged food. These relaxed primitive people all seemed to have one bowel movement within 20 to 30 minutes after each major meal that they ate. They just squat, it rapidly comes out within a minute, and they are done. No library of magazines, no squeezing, straining, grunting, meditation or prayer. It just came out effortlessly. They seem to average between 2 and 4 bowel movements a day or 14 to 28 bowel movements a week compared to the average American's bowel habit of 1 bowel movement every 3 to 5 days or 2 to 3 bowel movements a week. I figured this puts the Average American about 70,000 bowel movements short in their lifetime!

NORMAL CONSISTENCY

The consistency of your bowel movements should be soft and unformed like peanut butter or soft serve frozen ice cream. Occasionally they can be a bit chunky depending on what you ate and how well you chewed it, but in any case they should NOT be formed and they should be light in color. I remember as a kid my dad only went once a week on Sundays. He would take the entire Sunday paper in the bathroom and be in there for hours. When he came out the room smelled like someone died. I would then take my place at the throne after him and squeeze hard for my once a week bowel movement. Eventually I would blast out some small black balls as hard as granite. My dad would come into the bathroom to wipe me, but my fecal matter was so dry and hard there was nothing on the toilet paper. I remember my dad remarking, "Now that's a good poop, no wiping, like it's wrapped in cellophane" and I would leave for a week thinking I did a good job.

SIGNS OF CONSTIPATION

If you need a library in your bathroom, you know, like a stack of magazines on the hamper, then you are constipated. If you drink coffee, well, if you stop, you will also probably stop having bowel movements too.

DR. SCHULZE'S INTESTINAL DETOXIFICATION PROGRAM

MY PATIENTS TAUGHT ME THE POWER OF COLON CLEANSING

Like any great egomaniac student in herbal college, I wanted to develop very intricate and detailed herbal formulae. These formulae would be very difficult to make and could only be made from very exotic and rare herbs found only in the rainforest or in the Himalayas. And of course these formulae would be extremely effective for treating very specific diseases. I was going to find the herbal cure for Cancer...

Thank God my great teachers deeply ingrained in me that before I could embark on any of my disease-specific, smart-bomb herbal fantasies, I must get my patients on a good health program, first things first. First I needed to get them to follow the basics for a month or two, the basics being what I now refer to as my Foundational Programs, the foundations of health: a good clean and wholesome food program, thorough bowel cleansing and detoxification, immune boosting, exercise and positive emotional work. I knew that there was no replacement for these basics.

By doing so I unknowingly destroyed my fancy, disease-specific herbal formulae dream because approximately 80% of my patients, regardless of what was wrong with them, regardless of how long they had been sick, got more than relief. THEY GOT WELL! Just from bowel cleansing! When I added the other foundational programs, over 90% got well with no specific treatment at all. So much for my trips to Tibet.

You heard right. The vast majority of my patients got well and recovered from their diseases without ANY specific treatment. All they did was make some common sense lifestyle changes, including cleansing the bowel, and they were healed. My patients, having the nerve to get well before I was ready, ended all my dreams of discovering herbal cures for the afflictions of mankind and turned me into the common sense herbal country doctor that I am today.

NEVER, NEVER, NEVER UNDERESTIMATE THE POWER OF COLON CLEANSING

As I said, 80% of my patients' symptoms were gone just after they did a thorough bowel cleansing. When I ran my clinic, new patients were often upset when I told them we had to start with a thorough colon cleansing. What they wanted was my secret energy pill, or youth pill, or something to make their insomnia, infertility, back spasms, headaches, diabetes, arthritis, whatever, miraculously go away.

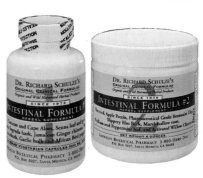

Natural Healing is NOT about temporary, quick fixes or pills to mask symptoms. It is NOT about cutting, poisoning and burning out disease. That's what medical doctors do. When you take that approach, often out of nowhere, your disease returns with a vengeance, much worse the second time around.

Natural Healing is about getting to the root cause of disease and illness, correcting it, and then building a healthy lifestyle so your body can do its' best healing possible. Then you can enjoy a long, healthy and energetic life.

MY PATIENTS THOUGHT I WAS FATHER SCHULZE, NOT DR. SCHULZE.

Most of my patients came into my clinic with a very guilty conscience regarding their lifestyle. They wanted to repent their sins of junk food and debauched living. They thought I could just wave my hands over them and have them say a few Hail Tofu's and everything would be OK. Well, it's not quite that simple. Most had already tried some kind of detox on their own, with either no results, or bad results.

Everyone nowadays is selling a quick detox or a 24 hour detox or some instant detox in a glass. There are a few problems here.

First, don't fool yourself. It takes most of us 20 or 30 years of rough and tough living before we develop a disease. So you're not going to heal yourself in 24 hours.

Secondly, I made my patients EARN the right to do a detox program. The reason for this is simple. When you start any detoxification program, what happens is that you dislodge and dissolve poisons and toxins that have built up in your fat and muscle cells and in various organs. During an effective detox, when these wastes are dissolved they are deposited into your colon for rapid elimination from your body. If you are constipated, or not having regular frequent bowel movements, these poisons sit there, can re-absorb and make you really sick. This is why many people who undertake a detox program without first making sure their colon is working feel weak, shaky, nauseous, headachy or HORRIBLE. I had patients that literally almost died doing intensive detoxification programs with hot saunas, gallons of juices, herbs, whatever, but hadn't had a bowel movement in weeks and the detoxification almost killed them.

This is why BEFORE you even think about any intensive detoxification program, THE COLON MUST BE ACTIVELY WORKING AND CLEAN!

FIRST THINGS FIRST!

This is worth repeating. The first step in any health program, especially BEFORE any blood and lymphatic cleansing or detoxification program, is to cleanse and detoxify the bowel. You must make sure it is working frequently and effectively and also make sure all of the old, toxic fecal material is out of the colon. Then you will enjoy an effective detoxification program, feel great while you're doing it and get the most out of it.

MY INTESTINAL DETOXIFICATION PROGRAM

THIS PROGRAM IS _VERY_ _EASY!_

Over 100,000 people worldwide have used this program to end their constipation, cleanse their colon, detoxify their

body and heal and prevent colon disease. It's easy and only takes a few minutes a day.

If you have never cleaned out your bowel and done an Intestinal Detoxification Program, CONGRATULATIONS! This is a great start to a new healthier life. As I said at the top, this program is Very Easy!

AN IMPORTANT TIP ABOUT INTESTINAL FORMULA #1

If you are like the majority of people and your bowel has not worked well most of your life, remember, Rome wasn't built in a day. Even if you have been extremely constipated all of your life, DO NOT try to fix yourself overnight. If you overdose and start off taking a dozen capsules of Intestinal Formula #1 you may learn the laws of jet propulsion, have a bad experience, or a messy one, and then stop doing the program. DON'T TORTURE YOURSELF! Be patient and start with only one capsule and increase by only one capsule daily as needed until your bowel is working.

ANOTHER IMPORTANT TIP ABOUT INTESTINAL FORMULA #1

If you have been constipated, especially if you have been for years, your bowel may not work perfectly at first. Just imagine if you had an old car in your garage that you hadn't started in years. The first time you go to start the engine it will shake, rattle and roll and smoke, backfire, make exploding noises, maybe even shoot flames out the carburetor. Then after about 15 minutes it will start running smoother, once it is warmed up. Your bowel is the same. If it hasn't worked properly in years, you may notice a little gas, or slight cramping, or even an occasional backfire. Do not be alarmed. This is usually caused by old fecal matter that is being flushed out and will subside usually within a few days. There are many herbs in the formula to reduce the chances of this happening, but if this occurs, KEEP GOING and continue to use the formula.

INTESTINAL FORMULA #2 IS ALSO VERY EASY

Occasionally a patient would say to me, "I can't drink this black drink" or "Isn't this program a bit radical?" GIVE ME A BREAK. WHAT TOTAL WIMPS! This drink might be black in color but it doesn't taste black. In fact, what little taste it does have is pleasant, especially if you are using diluted juice. And as far as radical, at what point did we start believing the lying medical doctors and start thinking that taking God's and Nature's healing gifts are radical? I'll tell you radical. Radical is when you develop colon disease and the doctors shove a colonoscope THREE FEET up your ass and then start burning and cutting off tumors on the inside of your bowel . . . . then you'll wish you had taken this formula. So don't you dare give me any damn radical crap and drink your drink, AND SMILE!

MY <u>TWO WEEK</u> INTESTINAL DETOXIFICATION PROGRAM

DAY #1: Start with one capsule of Intestinal Formula #1 during or just after dinner. This works best when mixed with food.

DAY #2: This morning you could notice an increase in your bowel action and in the amount of fecal matter that you eliminate. The consistency could also be softer. If you do NOT notice any difference in your bowel behavior today, or the difference wasn't dramatic, then tonight increase your dosage by 1 capsule. You can continue to increase your dosage every evening by one capsule until you notice a dramatic difference in the way your bowel works. Your goal is to increase your dosage until you are having 2-3 bowel movements a day. It has taken most of us years to create a sluggish bowel so let's be patient for a few days and increase by ONLY ONE capsule each day.

DAYS 3-7: Again, your goal is to be having at least two bowel movements each day, if not three. The average healthy person should achieve 2–3 bowel movements a day using this formula within this first week. If you don't, continue to take your Intestinal Formula #1 until you do. There is no race here to get to Intestinal Formula #2. Take your time and make sure your colon is working well, even if it takes a few weeks or a month.

WEEK #2: At the beginning of week two, or whenever your colon is working as described above, you may start using the Intestinal Formula #2. You will take this formula 5 times each day beginning in the morning. Start 1/2 hour after your morning nutritional drink, mix 1 heaping teaspoon of Intestinal Formula #2 powder with 8 ounces of diluted juice. It mixes best if you put a little liquid in the bottom of a small jar, then add your heaping teaspoon of Intestinal Formula #2. Then add the rest of the liquid and shake it vigorously. I drink it right out of my mixing jar, down the hatch, it takes only a minute, DONE. Do the same 1/2 hour before lunch, between lunch and dinner, 1/2 hour before dinner and 1 hour before bed, so that you are consuming a total of 5 heaping teaspoons each day.

DR. SCHULZE DESCRIBES HIS INTESTINAL FORMULAE

Intestinal Formula #1
(Cathartic Formula)

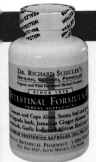

Botanical Ingredients: *Curacao and Cape Aloe leaf, Senna leaves and pods, Cascara Sagrada aged bark, Barberry rootbark, Ginger rhizome, Garlic bulb and African Bird Pepper.*

Therapeutic Action: This stimulating tonic is cleansing, healing and strengthening to the entire gastro-intestinal system. It stimulates your peristaltic action (the muscular movement of the colon) and over time strengthens the muscles of the large intestine. It halts putrefaction and disinfects, soothes and heals the mucous membrane lining of your entire digestive tract. This herbal tonic improves digestion, relieves gas and cramps, increases the flow of bile which in turn cleans the gall bladder, bile ducts and liver, destroys Candida Albicans overgrowth and promotes a healthy intestinal flora. It also destroys and expels intestinal parasites, increases gastro-intestinal circulation and is anti-bacterial, anti-viral and anti-fungal. Continue to use this formula until you are having at least 1 bowel movement each day for every meal you eat. Between 2 and 4 bowel movements a day is normal. Considering all the disease and death we have because of retained fecal matter, I wouldn't worry about taking too much of this formula.

Patient Type A: The sluggish bowel type. This formula is for 97% of my patients, the ones who need help getting their bowel working more frequently. You must use this herbal formula every day to keep your bowels very active.

Dosage: Start with only 1 capsule of this formula during or just after dinner. This formula works best when taken with food or juice. The next morning you should notice an increase in your bowel action and in the amount of fecal matter that you eliminate. The consistency should also be softer. If you do not notice any difference in your bowel behavior by the next day, or if the difference was not dramatic, then that evening increase your dosage to 2 capsules. You can continue to increase your dosage every evening by one capsule until you notice a dramatic difference in the way your bowel works. There is no limit. Some people have even needed over 30 capsules to get their bowel working. It has taken most of us years to create a sluggish bowel, so let's be patient for a few days and increase by only 1 capsule each day.

Patient Type B: The irritated bowel type. This only applied to a small percentage of my patients. These are the exceptions to the rule, those with bowels that move too often (more than 3 times a day.) This includes those with Colitis, Irritable Bowel Syndrome, Crohn's disease, etc... If your bowels are irritated, hot or working too frequently, skip this formula and go to Intestinal Formula #2.

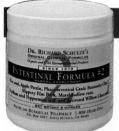

Intestinal Formula #2

(Drawing and Detoxifying Formula)

Botanical Ingredients: *Flax seed, Apple Fruit Pectin, Pharmaceutical Grade Bentonite Clay, Psyllium seed and husk, Slippery Elm inner bark, Marshmallow root, Fennel seed and Activated Willow charcoal.*

Therapeutic Action: This cleansing and soothing formula is to be used in conjunction with Intestinal Formula #1. This formula is a strong purifier and intestinal vacuum. This formula draws old fecal matter off the walls of your colon and out of any bowel pockets. It will remove poisons, toxins, parasites, heavy metals such as mercury and lead and even remove radioactive material such as Strontium 90. This formula will also remove over 3,000 known drug residues and toxic chemicals. Its mucilaginous properties will soften old hardened fecal matter for easy removal and make it an excellent remedy for inflammation in the intestines such as diverticulitis or irritable bowel. Many patients discovered that this formula also removed their colon polyps. This formula is an antidote for food poisoning and other types of poisoning. Therefore, I always have it with me when I travel.

Before beginning Intestinal Formula #2, your bowels should be moving at least 2 to 3 times a day or at least once for each meal you eat. Continue using Intestinal Formula #1 until this is achieved.

Dosage:

• Take Intestinal Formula #2 five times a day.

• Mix one heaping teaspoon of Intestinal Formula #2 powder with 8 ounces of juice or distilled water in a jar with a lid. Shake vigorously and drink immediately. Take anytime during the day, just be sure to allow about 30 minutes before or after meals, juices or taking your tinctures.

• Helpful hint: Put a small amount of water in your jar first. Then add the powder and shake. Then add more water. This keeps the powder from sticking to the jar, making it easier to clean.

• This formula contains bentonite clay and may be binding. Patient Type A's (defined under Intestinal Formula #1 on page 99) may need to increase dosage by one of the Intestinal Formula #1. Type B's may need to take one Intestinal Formula #1 in the evening if you find you are a little constipated.

HELPFUL HINT #1: Drink plenty of pure water, herb teas and diluted fruit juices during this two-week colon cleanse. A good amount is a minimum of 64 ounces to 128 ounces of liquid each day. This makes the program more effective.

HELPFUL HINT #2: Once you begin taking the Intestinal Formula #2, keep taking your Intestinal Formula #1 as usual, but increase the dosage you discovered the first week by 1 additional pill. If you feel a bit bound by the IF #2 you can increase your dosage of the IF #1 even more. It is helpful to drink more liquid after each dose of Intestinal Formula #2, at least 8 more ozs.

HELPFUL HINT #3: My audio tape, **Dr. Schulze Answers Your Questions, Volume #1,** has many, many answers to the most commonly asked questions, concerns and problems that my patients asked about my Intestinal Formulae #1 and #2 and my Intestinal Detoxification Program. Call **1-800-HERBDOC** and just ask for your free copy, it's on me.

6 CHAPTER SIX

CLEANSING AND DETOXIFICATION

If you want to be healthy and stay healthy, you need to flush out your Liver & Gallbladder and Kidneys & Bladder . . . . and do it regularly!

WHY SHOULD I?

We all know that taking our cars in for a checkup and changing the oil and the air filter and tuning the engine and rotating the tires makes the car last longer. Well, it's the same principle at work here. We can't expect to put a couple of hundred thousand miles on our body and never do any maintenance or change the oil. That just won't work. I want you to get out of the American medical syndrome of breakdown and repair and stop paying a trillion dollars a year for this torture. That's the way the medical system in America is designed. Go ahead, live in ignorance of your health; burn the candle at both ends; party, party, party. And then when the engine explodes and you're leaking everywhere you get to rebuild the entire engine (coronary bypass surgery, cancer chemotherapy and kidney dialysis is expensive torture.) Preventive maintenance is a lot cheaper and a lot more fun.

FACTS

- The American Society of Nephrology reports that over **40 MILLION** Americans have Kidney and Bladder INFECTIONS, IMPAIRMENT and DISEASE.

- Over **1/2 MILLION** Americans will have their constipated gallbladders carved out of their bellies <u>this year</u>!

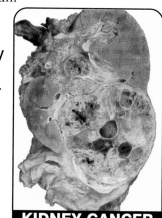

KIDNEY CANCER

- **Viral Hepatitis** *(liver inflammation)* has reached **Epidemic** proportions.

- Even the Food and Drug Administration has warned that there are over **50** different known **poisons** and **toxic substances** just in the average **American's grocery cart.** These chemicals combined cause **hundreds of different diseases** and eventually **KILL** you.

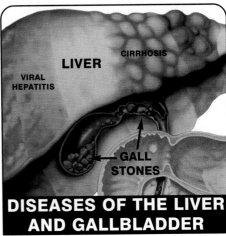

LIVER

CIRRHOSIS

VIRAL HEPATITIS

GALL STONES

DISEASES OF THE LIVER AND GALLBLADDER

HOW TO DO IT?

DIRECTIONS FOR DR. SCHULZE'S 5 DAY CLEANSING AND DETOXIFICATION PROGRAM

I created my 5 Day Cleansing and Detoxification Program as an entry level cleanse for all of my patients.

As discussed on the previous page, after my patients started taking their SuperFood on a regular basis and then did my Bowel Detoxification Program, and their bowel was working normally, it was then time to do their first detoxification program. If you are ill, you can start this 5 Day Program IMMEDIATELY! You don't have to do the Bowel Detoxification Program first, just add the Intestinal Formula #1 to the following program.

This program is an easy cleanse that ANYONE can do.

Come on friends, don't take this program *(or life, for that matter)* too seriously. Just do it--jump right in! Next Monday sounds like a good time to start to me, and if it's already Tuesday, how about a 4 Day Cleanse? LOOK, any of you out there who think that this might be a little inconvenient or cramp your busy lifestyle, well, all I can tell you is that once people end up in the hospital, under the knife, they wish they would have done it 20 times. But more importantly, everyone should experience a few days of a juice flush and a few days on raw foods. For my patients, this program turned their health and their life around.

I give you my guarantee that you will feel physically better, more alive and more energetic after 5 days on this program. Also, you will feel better about yourself and your life too! And a few of those aches, pains and disease symptoms you had...WILL BE GONE!

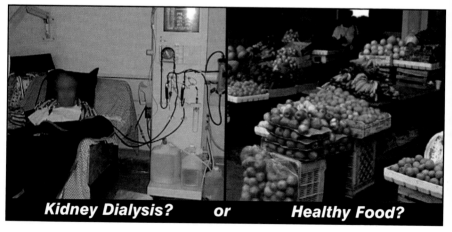

Kidney Dialysis?   or   **Healthy Food?**

IT'S YOUR CHOICE!

DR. SCHULZE'S
5 DAY CLEANSING AND DETOXIFICATION PROGRAM

THE PROGRAM IS 2 DAYS OF A PURIFYING RAW FOOD PROGRAM AND 3 DAYS OF A JUICE FAST.

HOW TO START YOUR FLUSH

YES, I designed my **5 Day Cleansing and Detoxification Program** to be done during the week, at work or during your regular weekly routine. Look, nobody wants to do a cleanse or detox on the weekend, and usually if you are silly enough to plan it that way, the phone rings, friends or relatives call, and the next thing you know, you've blown it. Weekend fun, friends, parties – eating is a big part of all of this. During the week you are very busy at work. You can do this program at work and <u>you will hardly even notice that you've done it</u>. IT WILL FLY BY. You might even set an example for a few of your co-workers, who would be nicer with their Livers & Kidneys cleaned out too.

STEP 1: Upon arising drink 8 oz. of distilled or purified water.

STEP 2: Next prepare and drink either the **Liver/Gall Bladder Flush, Liver/Gall Bladder Formula, Detoxification Tea** and **D-TOX Formula.**

OR

The **Kidney/Bladder Flush, Kidney/Bladder Formula, Kidney/Bladder Tea** and **D-TOX Formula.**

STEP 3: One hour later drink your **SuperFood Morning Nutritional Drink.**

STEP 4: Continue with the **Food Juice Program** as outlined next.

STEP 5: Remember to drink either the **Liver/Gall Bladder Formula** and **Detoxification Tea** *OR* **Kidney/Bladder Formula** and **Kidney/Bladder Tea** 2 more times during the day and **D-TOX Formula** 4 more times during the day.

Fresh fruit or vegetable juice is the best way to get your vitamins, minerals and other essential nutrients. They are also very important for cleansing and detoxification.

THE LIVER FLUSH
AND WHAT IT DOES

The main cause of Liver and Gall bladder disease is an overworked liver that is overloaded with toxins and poisons from our food, water and air and also from taking drugs, drinking alcohol and eating too much animal food. All of these cause the liver and gall bladder to be overloaded and subsequently congested, causing you to get sick. **This is the cause of almost all Liver and Gall bladder disease and also the cause of many seemingly unrelated diseases, even cancer, and these are the things that you need to STOP.**

The Liver and Gall bladder Flush Drink and Herbal Formulae stimulate the liver to produce more bile and get the bile moving through the Gall bladder and ducts. This action unblocks and unconstipates the Liver and Gall bladder and even dissolves and removes gall stones. **This is what will clean, detoxify and heal your Liver and Gall bladder and what you need to START.**

LIVER FLUSH DRINK

Mix the following in a blender:

During Spring or Summer, mix 8 ounces of fresh orange juice or better yet a citrus juice combination (1 lemon or 1 lime and enough orange, grapefruit or tangerine juice to make 8 ounces).
During Fall or Winter mix 8 ounces of fresh apple or grape juice or an apple/grape combination with:

- **8 ounces distilled or purified water.**
- **1-5 cloves of garlic (start with 1 and increase daily.)**
- **1-5 tablespoons of organic virgin cold-pressed olive oil (start with 1 and increase daily.)**
- **1 piece of fresh ginger root (about 1 inch long.)**
- **Don't chop the garlic or peel the ginger, just throw everything in the blender and liquify it. It only takes me 60 seconds to make my Liver Flush in the morning. Drink the flush down in 2-3 minutes, don't sip it.**
- 15-20 minutes after drinking your Liver Flush, drink 2 cups of previously prepared DETOXIFICATION TEA.
- Put 2 droppersful of my LIVER/GALL BLADDER FORMULA in each cup of tea (consume total of 4 droppersful) or have the tonic separately in an ounce of water.
- Finally take 3 droppersful of my D-TOX FORMULA. This formula is my strongest tasting so you can put it in a little grape juice if you wish.
- Repeat the same dosage of the LIVER/GALL BLADDER FORMULA & DETOXIFICATION TEA 2 more times during the day & D-TOX FORMULA 4 more times during the day.

THE LIVER FLUSH
SHOPPING LIST

Take this shopping list to the store with you and get these ingredients and you will be set up to do my entire 5-Day Liver Cleansing and Detoxification Program!

15-20 organic juice Oranges
(It is important to use organic when you're flushing because you don't want to put toxic, poisonous insecticides and pesticides into a drink that you are supposed to be cleaning your liver with, not poisoning it!)

5 organic Lemons and 5 organic Limes

2 bulbs of organic Garlic
(One bulb should do it, but why not have some extra garlic around?)

5 inches of fresh, organic Ginger Root
(Guys, come on, even if you have to spend two days going all over town to find organic, do your best so you are not putting poisons in your body.)

3 gallons of Distilled, Reverse Osmosis or Filtered Water (This will make enough for your Liver Flush Drink as well as the 2 1/2 gallons you'll need for your Detoxification Tea.)

1 24 oz. bottle of organic, extra-virgin cold-pressed Olive Oil

1 bottle of my Liver/Gallbladder Formula

1 bag of my Detoxification Tea

1 bottle of my D-TOX Formula

THE KIDNEY FLUSH
AND WHAT IT DOES

The Kidney and Bladder Flush and my Kidney and Bladder Herbal formulae have many healing benefits for your Urinary System.

First, just by consuming all the liquid you are literally flushing the Kidneys out. Just by urinating more you can remove infections and stones in the Kidneys and Bladder. This is very important, especially first thing in the morning, since your Kidneys have been sleeping and dormant all night long. In the morning you most likely have a higher bacteria count and higher level of sediment in your Kidneys than at any other time.

The citrus juices in the Kidney Flush not only supply you with needed electrolytes, but will alkalize your blood, which is proven to dissolve uric acid crystals and even Kidney stones. They also help to flush out mucous and are diuretic, making you urinate more.

KIDNEY FLUSH DRINK

Mix the following in a blender:

- **Juice of 1 lemon & 1 lime.**
- **16 - 32 ounces of distilled or purified water.**
- **A pinch of CAYENNE POWDER or 5 - 20 drops of CAYENNE TINCTURE.**
- <u>Optional:</u> A small amount of maple syrup to taste.
- Consume this drink.
- 15-20 minutes after drinking your Kidney Flush, drink 2 cups of previously prepared KIDNEY/BLADDER TEA.
- Put 2 droppersful of my KIDNEY/BLADDER FORMULA in each cup of tea (consume a total of 4 droppersful) or have the tonic separately in an ounce of water.
- Finally, take 3 droppersful of my D-TOX FORMULA. This formula is my strongest tasting so you can put it in a little grape juice if you wish.
- Repeat the same dosage of the KIDNEY/BLADDER FORMULA & KIDNEY/BLADDER TEA 2 more times during the day & D-TOX FORMULA 4 more times during the day.

The citrus juices contain citric acid. Apple cider vinegar contains acetic acid and can be used as a replacement if you cannot get good quality fresh citrus fruit. The apple cider vinegar must be raw, organic and unfiltered, like Bragg's or Spectrum. It will have the same action.

The Herbs in my Kidney/Bladder Formula and my Kidney/Bladder Tea have three major actions: Diuretic, Disinfectant and Dissolving. Herbs such as Uva Ursi Leaves, Juniper Berries, Corn Silk, Horsetail Herb, Parsley Leaf and Root, Carrot Tops, and others in the formula have been used for centuries as Diuretics (herbs that make you urinate more). Even today, most of these herbs are listed in medical and chemistry books for this action. Some of these herbs, like Juniper Berries and Uva Ursi Leaves, contain phytochemicals like volatile oils that are also powerfully disinfectant and destroy bacteria that live in your Kidneys and Bladder and therefore are healing for Kidney and Bladder Infections. Herbs like Hydrangea root and Gravel Root are famous for their ability to dissolve Kidney stones. So the Kidney and Bladder Flush, Kidney/Bladder Formula and Kidney/Bladder Tea make you urinate more, disinfect the Kidneys and Bladder and dissolve and flush out any sediment before it turns into rocks. And if you already have rocks, it starts breaking them down and dissolving them.

DIRECTIONS FOR HERB TEA

Put 6 tablespoons of **Detoxification Tea** or **Kidney/Bladder Tea** into 60 ounces of distilled water. Be sure to use only stainless steel or glass cookware. Let the tea sit in the water overnight. In the morning heat up to a boil, reduce heat and let simmer for 15 minutes (Detoxification Tea) or 1 minute (Kidney/Bladder Tea.) Strain the herbs, do not discard them, let the tea cool a bit, but use it hot. This will give you enough tea for your 6 cups for the day. Put the used herbs back into the pot, add 3 tablespoons of fresh herbs and 60 ounces of distilled water. Let sit overnight and repeat whole process. Keep adding new herbs to old ones for 3 days, then discard all herbs and start over. This is a great-tasting addition to your cleansing program. It will flush your system of toxins, acid and mucous while giving you concentrated amounts of minerals.

POTASSIUM BROTH RECIPE

This is a great-tasting addition to your cleansing program. It will flush your system of toxins, acid and mucous while giving you concentrated amounts of minerals.

Fill a large pot with 25% **potato** peelings, 25% **carrot** peelings and whole chopped **beets**, 25% chopped whole **onions** and **garlic,** 25% whole chopped **celery** and **dark greens.** Add hot peppers to taste. Add enough distilled water to just cover vegetables and simmer on very low temperature for 1-4 hours. Strain and drink only the broth, put the leftover vegetables in your compost. Make enough for two days, refrigerate leftover broth. Use only Organic vegetables! We do not want to consume any toxic, immune-suppressive insecticides, pesticides or inorganic chemical fertilizers while we are on a detoxification program.

My broth will flush you out and build you up. Start it now!

FOOD & JUICE ROUTINE
WHILE ON DR. SCHULZE'S 5 DAY CLEANSING AND DETOXIFICATION PROGRAM

DAY #1 AND #5

Breakfast: If you're hungry before lunchtime you may have fruit, diluted fruit juice and fruit smoothies. Stop all fruit and fruit juice at least 1 hour before lunch. It's best while on this program not to mix fruits and vegetables.

Lunch: For lunch you can have fresh raw vegetable juices, raw vegetables alone or in salads, sprouts, potassium broth, and herb teas. You may use dressings for your salads and vegetables if you like, using olive oil, avocado, raw apple cider vinegar, lemon juice, garlic, onions, and any herbs and spices.

Afternoon snacks: Raw vegetables, raw vegetable salads, diluted vegetable juices, sprouts, potassium broth, and herb teas. All vegetable foods and juices must be stopped by 6pm.

Dinner: Diluted fruit juices, fruit, fruit smoothies, fruit salads & herb teas.

DAY #2, #3, AND #4

Now we begin the 3-day fast. Consume at least 1 gallon (128 ounces) of liquid a day. That's eight 16-ounce servings a day. If you get hungry, DRINK MORE LIQUID!!!

Mornings: Start with water, your morning flush, herbal teas/tonics and your morning SuperFood drink.

Mid-mornings: Diluted fruit juices, herb teas and water until noon.

Afternoons: Diluted vegetable juices, potassium broth, herb teas and water until evening.

Evenings: Diluted fruit juice, herb teas and water in the evening.

DAY #5

Day #5 is the day you will be breaking your fast. Your food program will be the same as day #1. Breaking your fast is a very important part of this program. Chew your food slowly and mix each mouthful with plenty of saliva. Eat until you are satisfied, not full. You can always eat more later if you are still hungry. Chew everything to a liquid pulp.

DR. SCHULZE DESCRIBES HIS 5-DAY CLEANSING FORMULAE

Liver/Gallbladder
ANTI-PARASITE FORMULA

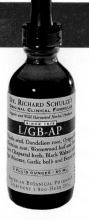

Botanical Ingredients: *Milk Thistle seed, Dandelion root and leaf, Oregon Grape root, Gentian root, Wormwood leaf and flower, Black Walnut hulls, Ginger rhizome, Garlic bulb, and Sweet Fennel seed.*

Therapeutic Action: The herbs in this formula are famous for their ability to **stimulate, cleanse and protect the liver and gallbladder and rid the body of parasites.** Milk Thistle has certain chemicals that bind to and coat liver cells. These phytochemicals not only heal previous liver damage, but also protect the liver from future damage. Oregon Grape rootbark, Gentian root, Wormwood leaves and Dandelion root are all classic bitter liver tonic herbs. These herbs not only stimulate digestion, but also stimulate the liver to excrete more bile, which in turn cleans both the liver and gallbladder. If you have been exposed to any toxic substances, had constipation, eaten large amounts of animal food or drank alcohol or other harmful beverages, this formula is for you. It is also beneficial if you have had high cholesterol, blood fats or any family history of liver or gallbladder problems. Many believe that anyone who has cancer or any immune dysfunction had a weak, congested liver to begin with. Even if a person has had their gallbladder removed these herbs will still be effective to clean the liver and bile ducts. The Black Walnut hulls, Wormwood and Garlic are strong **ANTI-PARASITICAL** plants. Parasite infestation is a fact of life. One cubic inch of beef can have over 1,000 living parasite larvae waiting to hatch in your body. Over 65% of fresh fish tested had toxic levels of bacteria and parasites. Chicken is even worse. I've had hundreds of patients expel bowls full of intestinal parasites, tape worms over 30 FEET LONG and also cellular parasites with these formulae. It works

best if used in conjunction with both **Intestinal Formulas #1 and #2.**
Use if parasites are suspected, or if there has been a history of bowel
problems, constipation, eating of animal products, prolonged illness,
disease and degeneration.

Dosage During the 5 Day Cleansing and Detoxification
Program: Add 2 droppersful to each cup of Detoxification Tea you
will drink. In the morning after your Liver/Gallbladder Flush you are
instructed to have 2 cups of Detoxification Tea 15 minutes after doing
your Liver/Gallbladder Flush, so that is a total of 4 droppersful after
your Liver/Gallbladder Flush. If you want you can have your tea
without this tonic, and consume it separately, 4 droppersful in 1 ounce
of water, at the same time as you drink the tea. Repeat having 2 cups of
Detoxification Tea and 4 droppersful of Liver/Gallbladder & Anti-
Parasite Formula 2 more times during the day.

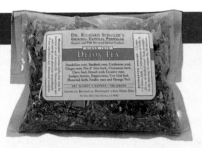

Detox Tea

Botanical Ingredients: *Roasted
Dandelion root, Burdock root, Pau
d'Arco inner bark, Cinnamon bark,
Cardamon seed, Licorice root, Fennel seed,
Juniper berries, Ginger root, Clove buds,
Black Peppercorns, Uva Ursi leaves, Horsetail herb, Orange peel and Parsley root.*

Therapeutic Action: This tea has numerous health benefits. First,
it is based on an ancient East Indian digestive tea formula. Over the
years in my clinic I have seen my patients eat almost anything and
survive, if they drank a cup of this tea before, during, or after the meal.
**It is a stimulant to the entire digestive process, especially the
stomach during the first stages of digestion. This tea also mildly
cleanses the blood, skin, liver and gallbladder and is the perfect tea
to use after the liver flush.** It flushes out the bile and fats from your
duodenum that the liver flush purged from your liver and gallbladder.
It is also a mild diuretic and disinfectant to the kidneys and bladder
and will cause you to urinate more within an hour after ingestion.

This tea is also an excellent coffee replacement. It is a hot beverage, dark in color, and tastes good. It's even better when a little pure maple syrup is added to the brew. It also increases your circulation, but has no caffeine. I used it in my clinic successfully for years to help people get off the coffee habit.

Dosage During the 5 Day Cleansing and Detoxification Program:

2 cups of tea consumed 15 minutes after doing your Liver/Gallbladder Flush. You should also have 2 more cups in the afternoon and 2 more cups in the early evening consuming a total of 6 cups of the Detoxification Tea each of the 5 days during this program.

D-TOX Formula

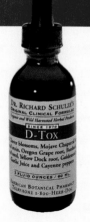

Botanical Ingredients: *Red Clover blossoms, Mojave Chaparral herb and resin, Oregon Grape root, Burdock root and seed, Yellow Dock root, Goldenseal root, Garlic juice, Lobelia seeds, Cayenne, and **a politically incorrect herbal base.***

Therapeutic Action: **This is a very powerful blood and lymph cleansing formula** and the one that I've used for years in my clinic. Every patient I treat and put on my **5-Day Cleanse** consumes one bottle of this formula during the week of this program.

This formula is based on the famous Hoxey Formula, Dr. Christopher's Red Clover Tonic formula and many similar formulae from around the world.

These herbs are famous for scrubbing the accumulated toxins and poisons out of the body's blood, fat and cells. As mentioned, it works best if used along with my **5-Day Cleanse.** When using this formula make sure to consume a gallon of water, juice and herbal tea each day.

After one of the late Dr. Christopher's arrests he was *instructed* never to use the word cancer again. In a private conversation I had with him regarding Red Clover Blossoms he said, "I just can't help myself, Red Clover is the antidote for cancer."

Chaparral is one of nature's most powerful anti-oxidants and has proven itself in the clinic to break up, destroy and dissolve all types of tumors.

The herbs in this formula are strong in taste, and very effective detoxifiers. Every patient I saw with chronic illness or degeneration used this formula with great success.

Dosage During the 5 Day Cleansing and Detoxification Program: You want to consume one entire bottle of my D-TOX Formula during your 5 Day Cleansing and Detoxification Program. This will be approximately 15 droppersful a day taken 3 droppersful 5 times a day. This is by far one of my most POWERFUL and STRONG TASTING herbal tonics. You will want to add your 3 droppersful to 1 ounce of strong apple or grape juice and knock it back. This is an herbal Jack Daniels, not a fine wine. Don't savor it. GET IT DOWN. You might even want a chaser.

Kidney/Bladder Formula

Botanical Ingredients: *Uva Ursi leaf, Juniper berries, Corn silk, Horsetail herb, Burdock root and seed, Parsley leaf and root, Pipsissewa leaf, and Goldenrod flower tops.*

Therapeutic Action: This tonic is both diuretic (increases the flow of urine) and disinfectant to the Kidneys, Bladder, and Urinary System. According to medical reports the herbs in this formula destroy the bacteria that cause Kidney and Bladder infections. More importantly, whenever I used this formula in my clinic, it cured every patient with a urinary tract infection, even after antibiotics had failed. It worked 100% of the time. This tonic formula works best if used along with the Kidney/Bladder Tea and the Kidney/Bladder Flush as directed in the 5 Day Cleansing and Detoxification Program.

Dosage during the 5 Day Cleansing and Detoxification Program: Add 2 droppersful to each cup of Kidney/ Bladder Herb Tea you will drink. In the morning after your Kidney/Bladder Flush you are instructed to have 2 cups of Kidney/Bladder Herb Tea 15 minutes after doing your Kidney/Bladder Flush Drink, so that is a total of 4 droppersful after your Kidney/Bladder Flush. If you want you can have your tea without this tonic, and consume it separately, 4 droppersful in 1 ounce of water, at the same time as you drink the tea. Repeat having 2 cups of Kidney/Bladder Herb Tea and 4 droppersful of Kidney/Bladder Formula two more times during the day.

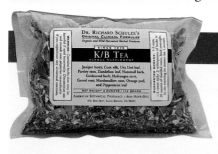

K/B Tea

Botanical Ingredients:
Juniper berries, Corn silk, Uva Ursi leaves, Parsley root and leaf, Carrot tops, Dandelion leaf, Horsetail herb, Goldenrod flower tops, Hydrangea root, Gravel root, Marshmallow root, Orange peel, and Peppermint leaf.

Therapeutic Action: Same powerful effect as the Kidney/ Bladder Formula above. This tea is most effective if used along with the tonic as directed in my 5-Day Cleanse. This formula also completely dissolves stubborn Kidney stones and calculi.

Dosage during the 5 Day Cleansing and Detoxification Program: 2 cups of tea consumed 15 minutes after doing your Kidney/Bladder Flush. You should also have 2 more cups in the afternoon and 2 more cups in the early evening consuming a total of 6 cups of the Kidney/Bladder Tea each of the 5 days during this program.

DR. SCHULZE
QUOTE: "Your body has a BLUEPRINT, a SCHEMATIC, of what perfect health is and is constantly trying to achieve this goal for YOU."

7 CHAPTER SEVEN

BREATHE DEEPER

Breathe deeper, to get more air into your lungs and to exhale more waste gas.

WHY SHOULD I?

Oxygen is the #1 most primary nutrient to every cell in your body. Deep Breathing is a powerful food for the body and also a powerful cleansing and detoxification aid.

FACTS

- You can go months without solid food. I have personally done that on extreme cleansing routines like my incurables program. I have had many patients that have gone half a year without any solid food and one patient that went an entire year.

- You can even go days without liquid, sometimes called a dry fast, and survive just fine. But you can only go a few minutes without breathing or you DIE!

- This simple fact proves that Oxygen is the #1 most primary nutrient to the human body. More than any food, more than any liquid. Without it, you are dead in just a matter of a few minutes.

- The American Lung Association states that smoking-related diseases claim an estimated 430,700 American lives each year. Smoking costs the United States approximately $97.2 billion each year in health-care costs and lost productivity. It is directly responsible for 87% of lung cancer cases and causes most cases of emphysema and chronic bronchitis.

- Even if you don't smoke, working next to, or living with, a smoker can kill you. There are an estimated 38,000 deaths due to second-hand smoke each year.

How To Do It?

IF YOU SMOKE TOBACCO, STOP HERE!

If you smoke put this book down and get yourself help. This is not some anti-smoking prejudice. I don't care if people smoke but one thing I know for sure is that you can't smoke and get healthy or be healthy, PERIOD.

So I don't care how you do it—just do it. Go to quit smoking groups; go to therapy; use the patch; use lobelia; get shocked with cattle prods, take drugs that make you puke if you smoke or get hypnosis or tie your damn hands behind your back. Whatever it takes, I really don't care, just stop smoking, because you cannot be well and smoke. It's impossible.

As I stated above, the most primary nutrient of your body is oxygen. You can go months without food; days without liquid or drinking water; but you can only go minutes—seconds—without air and oxygen. And then you die. Your brain dies. You're dead.

The act of smoking is the act of willfully and knowingly destroying the only organ in your body that digests and assimilates oxygen. It's not like if your lungs fail that your ears will start breathing for you. So by smoking you are clogging up the pores on the surface of your lungs with tar and slowly smothering yourself, slowly killing yourself. It is absolute unadulterated suicide and you cannot be well. <u>So if you still smoke, close this book now. You can't be well and smoke, so close the book</u>. When you stop I'll be here waiting for you. **<u>I never ever worked on a patient who smoked, ever.</u>** I threw every one of them out on their ass on their first visit to my clinic. They're not bad people. I even smoked as a kid and teenager for years, 2 to 3 packs a day. So I am not some virgin sex counselor preaching about what I haven't personally experienced. And believe me, I know how addicting tobacco is, but I am also not Jesus, and I can't perform some miracle to let you smoke and still be well. You cannot smoke and be well so you must quit smoking first and then come back to the book. And I will welcome you back with fanfare.

BEGIN ROUTINE DEEP BREATHING

This is really simple and fun. Just pick a time, anytime, when you wake up and are still in bed to when you are back in bed ready for sleep, or anytime in between. Obviously it is best to open the windows if you do this inside the house and get the freshest and cleanest air possible. Getting outside and even slow walking while doing this is optimum. Morning time in the country and even in big cities tends to be the cleanest air time. If you happen to be on the 30th floor of some building that has sealed windows and conditioned air, well, if possible get hepa air filters, ionizers, ozone generators, breathing dust masks, a gas mask, whatever, and clean up the air as best as possible. In most cases deep breathing of poor quality air is still better than shallow breathing it.

Now this isn't rocket science. Just start slow, rhythmic, deep breathing to drive air deeper into your lungs. Most people only use about the top third of their lungs and are what I refer to as shallow breathers. So open up and stick out your chest and take some slow deep breaths, hold them for a second and then do a complete, more forceful than usual exhale.

The absolute best way is to inhale through your nose and then exhale through your mouth. Most people breath this way naturally. I don't want you to become self-conscious or paranoid about your breathing but this is the proper and best way to breathe. Mouth breathers (meaning people that always inhale through their mouth) are absolutely not as healthy as nose breathers.

I told you about oxygen being the most primary nutrient to your body and that deep breathing was the best way to get more of it in. Deep breathing is also the best way to get more of your blood's waste gas (carbon dioxide) out of your body. If too much of this poisonous gas backs up and then builds up in your blood, it will make you sick, cause disease and eventually kill you. So deep breathing is not only the best way to let the good in but to get the bad out.

If you really want to get into it more you can go to a hatha yoga studio and tell them you are interested in pranayama or the yogic science of breathing. Most yoga studios teach some sort of breath work.

Some styles of yoga, like Swami Satchidinandas Integral Yoga, have it developed to such a science, like their three-part breath, that just the act of breathing is a powerful healing therapy. It is also an integral part of many traditional martial arts from Chi Gung to Karate's SanChin Breathing katas. Almost all traditional martial arts used some type of deep breathing to light the fire in the hara and build up internal energy called chi (Chinese), ki (Japanese), prana (Indian) and often translated as meaning Life Force.

Often when I would tell my patients to pay attention to their breath and maybe to go out and get lessons on breathing they would first look at me like I was some sort of quack. But after their first lesson, they thanked me.

But whether you decide to become an oxygen junky or you just pick 10 minutes a day to do your deep breathing, as Nike says, JUST DO IT.

BEYOND BREATHING

Like all of my other 20 tips, once you begin to let yourself play with them and are not being too serious, magic will start to happen.

Try breathing in through your nose and out through your mouth as I suggested above. But when you exhale, make an audible sigh or groan. Let the sound be determined as a reflection of you letting go of all of your physical, emotional or spiritual stress. At first it may sound a bit contrived. You might have to force yourself to pretend a bit at first. Some of us have had many more years of practice in the art of not expressing ourselves as others, but give it a go. Once you get the hang of it you will forget about this book, forget your embarrassment, forget your breathing and moaning and the next thing you may hear is the police knocking on your door thinking that someone is dying inside your house. You can tell them it's just the opposite.

BEYOND BEYOND BREATHING

There are even advanced therapies that take breathing far and beyond just getting a more complete breath and exhale. Re-birthing, which can now be referred to under many different names, is a therapy of deep, continual, rhythmic breathing which can send you into a deep state of self-awareness, even emotional catharsis and physical tetany. I used this therapy often in my clinic, under certain circumstances. I found it to be very beneficial to my patients. One reason was to just physically supercharge them with oxygen and chi, and to move energy within their body. Sometimes I used it to break them through blocked or stuck physical energy or crystallized emotional or spiritual issues. With the right therapist it can be a great healing tool. I am not suggesting that you need to go out and do it, nor am I suggesting you don't. I did feel it appropriate to tell you about it here.

So take a deep breath and . . . . another one . . . .and another one . . . .

DR. SCHULZE
QUOTE: "EVERYONE DIES, but not EVERYONE really LIVES."

8 CHAPTER EIGHT

STRETCHING, WALKING, MOVING

You must exercise every day.
Do whatever you can, but push yourself.
Increase the amount every day.
You should breathe hard and work up a sweat.
1 hour each day is to be your eventual goal.

WHY SHOULD I?

You've heard it before: If you rest you rust, and all that. But moving your body is not just exercise to be fit. Every function in your body depends upon your moving—everything. Your blood circulation, your lymphatic circulation, your nerve function, your digestion, assimilation, elimination, your brain—everything.

FACTS

- Over 50% of deaths due to chronic disease are caused by a sedentary lifestyle.

- Over 108 MILLION American adults (61%) are either obese or overweight.

- 50 MILLION are medically considered OBESE! That's over 25% of all adults.

- Women who engage in 'brisk' walking for one hour a day have
  20% less chance of Breast Cancer
  30% less chance of Heart Disease
  50% less chance of Diabetes.

- A study at the CDC, Center for Disease Control, estimated there are 88 million inactive Americans over the age of 15 years. If they would start moderate regular physical activity it would reduce annual medical costs by $76.6 BILLION.

HOW TO DO IT?

I want you to move every day for one hour, and I want you to sweat, bend and stretch. Yeah, walking, running, bending, stretching, dancing, sex—whatever. Just do it for an hour every day.

STRETCHING

I have converted a room of my house into an exercise and movement room. But before we even get there I want to tell you about my bedroom. It is a jungle of STRETCHING TOYS. First off I have one of those big inflatable stretching balls. It's at least 24" if not bigger and bright tie-dyed color. It looks absolutely ridiculous in the middle of my bedroom, I can't hide it anywhere and it looks like a gigantic kid's ball. It makes me laugh when I see it and almost cry when I lie all over it. It is an incredible, inexpensive and great stretching aid to open up your chest, stretch your spine and make your body supple.

Inversion is a wonderful way to temporarily give your body a break from gravity. It does you such good to take the pressure off of everything, from your spinal discs to your transverse colon. It is also a great way to get more blood up into your head and brain. I have used gravity boots for years to invert myself but I recently traded them in for a backswing type of device. Standing up, you strap yourself onto a cot or soft body board and lean back and you can become completely inverted, without as much stress on your ankles. Sure, you can also use a slant board, or put books under your bed posts. There are a lot of ways to get slanted and upside down so just do it.

What you are starting to hear from me is that I like toys. Wait a minute, what am I saying, I LOVE TOYS!

TOYS YIPEE!

I am a big lover and fan of toys, all kinds of toys. In case you forgot,

TOYS ARE FUN!

I have found with myself, and all of my patients, that if you are trying to start a new program, then buying some related toys will increase your chances of success **1000 times.** Don't make any new health program boring and torturous or you will end up quitting it faster than you started it. I quit anything **immediately** if I am not having fun. Toys make anything much more fun and interesting. So if you are a lazy ass like most of us, then buying some exercise-related toys will spark and keep your interest.

And don't be cheap with yourself, especially when you are creating this new healthy life. You are saving about $2,000 a day for every day that you keep yourself out of the hospital. Now you are doing the best things for yourself that you have done in years, maybe even your whole life, that will increase your health and life span, **so get out and buy some toys**.

You can spend the money now on fun things, or spend it later on coronary bypass surgery. It's your choice, but I chose the toys...

SUGGESTED TOYS

When doing fat burning or cardiac strengthening exercise, one toy that can keep you entertained is a heart/pulse monitor. There are various types of pulse monitors available for sale that can be very helpful to keep you in your fat-burn range during any exercise. Some, like the Polar, have a band that connects around your chest and a wristwatch. You set the heart rate that you want to achieve and maintain into the watch (it's easy) and then start moving. Running, Marching, Swimming (underwater is ok), whatever, this watch will monitor your pulse rate, it will even beep if you go out of your preset fat-burning range to alert you and keep you steady and it also keeps track of how many minutes and seconds you have maintained your fat-burn heart rate.

As I said there are various manufacturers of these pulse monitor devices and I have found them all to be good. I am just used to the Polar brand because I have been using one for a few decades.

Get yourself a great pair of walking or running shoes. You know that most of these shoes break down and go flat after about 6 months so don't go out for your first walk in a 5-year-old pair of broken down tennis shoes. Get some with some great spring in them and that look cool. My personal favorite is Nike, but there are many brands and many opinions. One suggestion: buy the pair that is just a little bit more outrageous looking than you would normally go for, because with this new body you are going to have, you will want to draw a little more attention and show it off, so take the leap now.

Get some workout clothes. I suggest getting them a little tighter, ones that show off your body more. This way you won't bullshit yourself after your first day of exercise that one day made a big difference and was all that you needed. Don't hide your fat when you exercise; flaunt it. It helps to keep you motivated and KEEP YOU GOING.

If you exercise inside your house in private, wear as little clothing as necessary, nothing if possible. Seeing your fat jiggle and wobble while you exercise, if you are fairly emotionally stable, can be a great motivational tool.

Another thing that I like is a cool baseball-type hat and don't forget to bend the brim so you don't look like a geek. Also, maybe a day pack or a belt fanny pack. The company Eagle Creek makes a lot of great fanny packs that are designed well and have lots of useful pockets. The company North Face makes what I think are the best day-type backpacks because they are contoured to fit your body better, have a waist belt, great padded shoulder straps and have lots of useful pockets.

If music or even my GET WELL Audio Tape turns you on and will keep you going, get a walkman or a Discman and some lightweight sports earphones. Actually they are more like ear plugs than headphones and the sports ones are yellow and won't short out as easy when you fill them with sweat or spill your Evian on them.

I could go on forever, but I think you get the point. GET TOYS to keep you motivated and having fun. They are worth 1000 times their cost in adding years to your life and keeping you out of the hospital.

OK, BACK TO STRETCHING...

One of the best stretching systems is Hatha Yoga. Contrary to what some believe it is NOT a religion. It may have been incorporated into some but in and of itself it is not. It is a scientific system of stretching, inversion practices, deep breathing, and many other things. All of the postures are designed to put pressure on certain organs like endocrine organs and various glands of the body and this promotes cleansing, detoxification and health building. It also increases your immune strength.

Being flexible not only ensures that you have a strong back, but flexible people live longer too. Start stretching today!

WALKING

Walking is so simple and at the same time a powerful healing tool. So I want you to walk more. I want you to walk where you would normally drive. If you take the bus to work, get off a few blocks too soon or too late and walk. If you take an elevator, get off a few floors too soon and take the stairs up to your office. No matter how you do it, WALK MORE.

And while you're walking, remember (chapter 7), deep breathing and breathe deeper. Get more air in and out of your lungs, which is going to get more oxygen in your bloodstream and in all the cells of your body. It's a great first step in getting healthy. And while you're out there walking, try some barefoot walking (see chapter 10). Go out into the grass or the beach or the woods and take your shoes off and actually touch the earth, the planet you live on. It will ground you. It will help you release built-up electrical energy that's in your body. Remember, your entire nervous system is run on electrical energy. Your heart beats on electrical impulses and you build up the static electricity. So get your shoes off and get in touch with the earth. GET WALKING AND GET BREATHING. It will change your life.

MOVING

FAT BURNING VS. HEART STRENGTHENING

The facts at the beginning of this chapter should motivate everyone to burn off a little extra fat. The best movements for burning fat off of your body are ones that keep your heart rate steadily above normal for a set period of time. This type of movement is most often called Aerobic exercise, which means increasing the use of the heart and lungs but is now used to refer to just about any exercise that keeps your pulse rate consistently and continuously above normal.

In other words, exercise like playing the board game monopoly, even though you may jump up and down occasionally for 2 to 3 hours, is not STEADY enough. Other sports that come into this category would be golf, tennis, baseball, football, even weightlifting, because they are on and off heart rate sports.

Sex can be rhythmic and steady and therefore aerobic, but since the average time it lasts in America still hasn't pushed the 3 minute envelope, this isn't LONG enough (see my Male and Female Sexuality GET WELL Newsletter).

What we need is a STEADY and LONG or CONTINUOUS movement that will keep your heart rate or pulse at a certain level for a certain amount of time.

HOW FAST FOR HOW LONG?

There are various ranges where you can keep your heart rate or pulse rate above normal and some of these ranges are known to be best for all around fitness. Other ranges are best for heart muscle toning, sometimes called the cardio ranges, and still other pulse ranges are most efficient for burning up fat.

The most simple way to discover your best heart or pulse range for fat burning is to take the number 220 and then subtract your age. Say you are 50 years old. Well, 220 minus 50 is 170. Now you take a percentage of this number. Most types of aerobic exercise keep the heart between 55% and 85% of this number. 55% is a good beginning range if you are out of shape but 65% is now considered by most exercise gurus to be the best fat burning range. 75% to 85% is considered to be the best cardiac conditioning range, BUT NOT THE BEST FAT-BURNING RATE.

So 65% of this number, the lower end of the range, is considered to be the best FAT-BURN pulse rate to maintain, so, using the following calculation, anyone can determine their best pulse rate to burn fat.

220 minus (age) times 65% = best FAT burn pulse rate.

220 minus (age) times 75% to 85% = best Heart Conditioning pulse rate.

It is necessary to keep fairly steady at this heart range for about 45 minutes to 1 hour.

HOW DO YOU KNOW IF YOU'RE IN THIS RANGE?

The easiest way is to just start moving, like walking fast, and after a few minutes check your pulse. Don't try it with a few fingers on the inside of your wrist like a nurse does in a hospital. You may find this hard to find and not easy when you are walking. Once you get moving, huffing and puffing and a sweat breaks, just grab yourself around your neck like you are trying to strangle yourself with one hand, but not quite as hard. Don't worry about trying to place your thumb and fingers on your carotid artery, just grab your neck and if you are moving enough you will easily feel your pounding pulse.

Next, if you do this with your right hand, look at the watch on your left hand, and count how many pulses you feel in a certain amount of time. Like how many pulses you count in 6, 10 or 15 seconds and then multiply them accordingly. You don't want to count for 30 seconds or a whole minute because this takes too long and will slow you down, and slow down your heart rate, which is exactly what you DON'T want to do.

Count your heartbeats in 6 seconds, multiply by 10, that equals your pulse.

Count your heartbeats in 10 seconds, multiply by 6, that equals your pulse.

Count your heartbeats in 15 seconds, multiply by 4, that equals your pulse.

NOTE: Generally speaking, if you can carry on a normal conversation and sound perfectly normal, you are not exercising aggressively enough. If you can hold a conversation but your voice stutters a bit and you gasp for air interrupting your speech occasionally, then you are roughly in the right fat-burn range. If you can't hold a normal conversation and you are gasping and huffing and puffing so much that you can't talk, then you are probably out of and above your fat-burn range.

WHAT TYPE OF EXERCISE IS BEST TO DO AND FOR HOW LONG?

Basically the best type of exercise is ANYTHING that you are willing to do that also keeps your heart rate steady in your best fat-burning range. The easiest and most available is walking. Yes, most of you, at least at first, should have no problem staying in your best fat-burning range by just *fast* walking. Running is usually not necessary. Walking is also a great way to deep breathe, get some fresh air and check out the neighborhood, and is low impact so you won't get extremely sore.

If you refuse to go outside or you live in Buffalo and it's winter (I can bitch, I grew up in Rochester), buy a treadmill. There are many types on the market. Or join a gym. I don't watch television ever, it is not a part of my life, except, when I get on a treadmill I find it so boring, I watch a little TV to catch up on the latest nauseating bad news or the latest demented reporting and catch a few commercials so I have something to write about in my Politically InCorrect column. You can also join a gym that has treadmills and exercise classes. Going to different exercise classes (keep them aerobic and fat burning) or finding a exercise buddy, or even hiring a personal trainer will also increase your chances of success.

The best amount of time to continue the movement for is about 1 hour. This gives you a few minutes to warm up to your target fat-burning pulse rate and a few minutes to cool down at the end and still get in at least 45 minutes of 65% fat burning range of aerobic exercise.

NOTE: If you are fat or out of shape or both and not used to this type or any type of exercise then it is best to start off easy. It won't be to your benefit to give yourself a heart attack trying to get healthy, so for the first 2 weeks just work your way up to my suggestions. Most importantly, you should be sweating. If you are not sweating, I don't care what the numbers say, you will not be burning fat.

BEYOND WALKING

Dance, Swim, Roll Around, Jump. Walk, Run, Hop like the freakin' Easter bunny, I don't care but get up off your lazy butt and start moving that thing or lose it.

The bottom line: moving your body makes you healthier and makes you live longer. It's not if you rest you rust, it's if you rest you DIE, so get out there and start moving.

DR. SCHULZE
QUOTE: "All disease is caused by some type of BLOCKAGE. Whether it's blood, lymphatic, nerve, nutritional, elimination, emotional, spiritual, whatever, FREE the blockage and the healing begins immediately."

9 CHAPTER NINE

WATER THERAPY (*HYDROTHERAPY*)

The fastest, strongest and most effective way to increase your blood and lymphatic circulation is the application of Hot and Cold Water.

WHY SHOULD I?

The cause of ALL disease is some type of BLOCKAGE! Something . . .blood supply, lymphatic fluid, nerve force, oxygen intake, nutrition assimilation, physical blockage, and even emotional and spiritual blockage. What I know is that when any area of your body gets sick and diseased, something is blocked off to it.

Blood carries oxygen and nutrition, brings <u>LIFE</u> to every cell and every organ in your body. When the blood is restricted to any area of the body, that area gets sick. If the blood gets blocked off, that area DIES!

FACTS

- **COLD** water applied to the surface of the body turns the skin white. This is because it contracts the surface skin, muscle and blood vessels and **pushes away** the surface blood volume deeper into your body.

- **HOT** water does the exact opposite. The skin turns red because **hot** water expands the surface skin, muscles and blood vessels and **draws** more blood to the surface of the body.

- By alternating **HOT** and **COLD** water to the surface of the body, you can increase your circulation in that area more than any other way. <u>**Increasing the circulation HEALS YOU FASTER. It's that simple**</u>.

HOW TO DO IT?

WHAT IS HYDROTHERAPY?

As a professional body worker using numerous physical therapies in my clinic, I witnessed the awesome power of touch in healing people. With the right person doing it, it's so powerful. Apply pressure, energy and consciousness to a person's body in the right way and the body, mind and spirit can change. Body work effects the breathing, the circulation and the temperature of the body. It moves the blood, lymphatic fluid and stimulates the nerves, and it can cause emotional catharsis and healing and so much more. Getting regular bodywork and different types of bodywork is HEALING!

Another powerfully healing physical *and emotional* therapy is hydrotherapy, simply meaning *water*therapy This miraculous healing therapy went out of *vogue* in America in the last century because it involved nudity, not because it didn't work. In fact it is still extremely popular in many other countries where the people live much longer and much healthier than they do in the United States.

All the natural healers of old used hydrotherapy in their clinics along with the herbs, the elimination and detoxification routines, the food programs, exercise and emotional and spiritual healing.

Nowadays people swallow a pill and expect a miracle, but true and lasting health doesn't come that cheap. Sometimes it takes a lot of dedication and a lot of hard work to be well, and Hydrotherapy was part of EVERY ONE OF MY PATIENT'S PROGRAMS and a big part of my *incurables* program.

John Harvey-Kellogg of Battle Creek, Michigan cured the incurables using water therapy, whole foods and body work. There was a great naturopathic doctor named Benedict Lust who came over to this country from Europe. Benedict Lust had a method he called the blood washing method where he kept you in **hot** and **cold** applications for eight hours straight. This treatment became world famous for its healing power and ability. Father Sebastian Kneipp was a healer from the late 1800's. His great book is not just an Herbal, although it does contain many pictures of herbs and how to use them. But many of these old Herbals and healing books also contained numerous chapters on hydrotherapy, including Father Kneipps'.

The great doctors' therapies and their books contained all types of water therapies, how to apply the water, what temperature of water to use, the force of the water and where to apply it. There would be hundreds of detailed pictures and drawings in each of these books describing the various methods.

Many, many years ago I wanted to investigate hydrotherapy so I went down to one of the last operating hydrotherapy clinics in the United States. (Now before you send me letters I know there are many spas across America but I am talking about powerful, 25 water treatment, kick butt hydrotherapy. Not a spa.) I wanted to experience the healing power of some of these great old treatments that were in this country years ago, before they were gone. I chose Hot Springs, Arkansas but was saddened to see that only one or two, I believe, of the original 12 were still in operation and none of them offered the intense hydrotherapy treatments that they did fifty or one hundred years ago.

When I walked up to this clinic what did I see? There were elderly people sitting all over the porch with their heads down, looking stunned, dazed and doped up, almost drooling on the floor. It looked more like a sanitarium for the brain dead, but I wanted to see what, if anything, they still offered.

So I went in and I said, "Give me the full hydrotherapy treatment, please". What did they do? They put me in a hot tub, made me drink **hot** water. Then they took me out and put me in a shower, and **cold** water jets hit me all over the body, then I went into another hot tub and a steam bath, then they put me in a room and they put hot packs and ice packs all over my body, and then laid me down in another bed for a few minutes to rest, then finally put me in a wheelchair and wheeled me out to the front, where I sat with all these other people staring at the floor with drool coming out of my mouth. Now I realized that these people were not brain dead, there was nothing wrong with them, they were RELAXED, PHYSICALLY BLISSED OUT, EMOTIONALLY AND SPIRITUALLY HEALED.

This is when I truly learned the SHEER POWER of HOT and COLD water and how it affects you, how it heals your body, mind and spirit. WOW, HYDROTHERAPY!

I felt more power in this 1 hour hydrotherapy treatment than in years of other therapies.

Thank God these hydrotherapy clinics still operate all over Europe. In Belgium, Luxembourg, France, Germany, Italy, even in what we think is conservative England, they exist. In fact, when I finish this book I am taking a few weeks off and going over to Europe for what I call a hydrotherapy vacation where I will visit many hydrotherapy clinics and *take the waters.*

HOT water sedates you, relaxes you, and while it's relaxing you it relaxes and loosen your muscles. It also brings all the blood in your body to the very surface, which is why your skin turns red.

COLD water does just the opposite; it stimulates you, it wakes you up. It contracts the muscles and it drives all the blood that's on the surface of your body into the deeper organs.

By alternating from **HOT** to **COLD** and then back to **HOT** again, you are bringing the blood to the surface of your body, then driving it back to the center core of your body, and then drawing your blood back to the surface again.

This is much more powerful and much faster at moving your blood than any massage, exercise or even the hottest cayenne pepper. Now just imagine if you did them all!

DR. SCHULZE'S HOT AND COLD HYDROTHERAPY ROUTINE

Just get into a nice warm shower (a blend of **HOT** and **COLD** water) for a few minutes and relax, then when you're ready, quickly turn the **HOT** water off all the way, and take that full blast of **COLD** water on your entire body, *everywhere,* especially the sick areas, and don't forget your head. It is also helpful to scream, yell, moan, cry, shake and do whatever comes naturally. Actually, what usually comes naturally is very little because we have had years of training in swallowing our emotional expression, so unload and scream.

After about 15 – 30 seconds, whatever you can stand, turn the **HOT** water back up slowly, take a few seconds, and turn it up to as hot as you can stand it. Make sure that it hits you everywhere again for about 15 seconds, even up to a minute if you can. Then immediately turn the hot water off all the way again.

If you understood me correctly you are only turning the **HOT** water on and off but you will be leaving the **COLD** water always running.

Once you get the hang of this I want you to do 7 repetitions of **HOT** and **COLD**, that's 7 **HOTS** and 7 **COLDS**.

If you do this **HOT** and **COLD** alternating hydrotherapy shower on or over any diseased area of your body, or on any sick area, any blockage, any pain, any cyst, boil, cancer, or physical injury along with the other programs in this book, the next thing you will know, your problem will be gone.

P.S. *Don't be stupid. If you have a history of any heart or circulatory disease, work your way into this program more slowly, using your good common sense.*

DR. SCHULZE
QUOTE:

"There are NO *incurable* diseases, NONE. If you are willing to take RESPONSIBILITY for yourself and your life, you can heal yourself of anything."

10 CHAPTER TEN

NATURAL CLOTHING

Wear cotton, wool, linen, silk and other natural fiber clothes

WHY SHOULD I?

Your skin actually breathes, and in order for your skin to breathe it can't be sealed shut. Imagine putting plastic wrap all over your body or sealing your body with a couple of coats of varnish. This could eventually kill you because **your skin has to breathe!**

FACTS

• Your skin is an amazing organ. It <u>absorbs nutritional substances,</u> <u>converts sunlight to vitamin D,</u> <u>has its own immune system</u> and **it can also eliminate up to 10 pounds a day in gases, liquid and semi-solids**.

• Synthetic fibers like polyester, nylon, lycra, and spandex don't breathe. They might make great wrinkle-free, wash and wear clothes, but they don't let air in and they don't let your skin's elimination out.

• Your body, in its normal course of metabolic function, creates electricity. What you wear on your feet can restrict this built-up excess electricity from getting out of your body. When not eliminated and discharged, this built-up electricity causes nervousness, anxiety, tension, insomnia and emotional and physical stress that can instigate disease.

HOW TO DO IT?

An often overlooked but important aspect of creating a new healthy life is having a clothing *makeover*. In other words, when you heal your disease you will also create a new healthy body, mind and spirit. Literally a new you!

In my clinic, many of the patients that came to see me were dying from their disease. In order for such sick patients to heal themselves naturally they had to change just about EVERY aspect of their life. Often after a few months on my programs most patients would have a sudden awareness. Often they would be lying on my examination table talking with me when all of a sudden they would *quickly* sit up, get a shocked and even anxious look on their face and exclaim, "I don't even know who I am anymore." I would often yell GOOD, because who you used to be was Cancer, or Heart Disease or Dying.

It was usually at this time I would suggest to my patients to take on a new name or an appearance change. I would have already made them wear natural fiber clothing, but at this point we would get fashionable.

Art Linkletter was right, people are funny. During life so many things seem to be so important: our hair style, our complexion, our appearance to others, what others think or clothing style. I am not saying that these things aren't important, but it is interesting that when all of a sudden we are faced with death, our whole outlook on life changes. I was very fortunate to have this near-death illuminating experience myself at the early age of 16. When facing death, what was important often seems trivial now. My patients would often remark, "I can't believe I even cared about that." And other things that we took for granted, like eating, breathing, laughing and sleeping now become very important.

Almost always, after a huge life-saving health turnaround, my patients would stop being so concerned with what others might think about them or their appearance. *Often this worry contributed to their disease in the first place.* Now they were finally ready to do what **they** wanted to do, maybe for the first time in their life, and this included WHAT THEY WANTED TO WEAR.

What I am telling you is that you don't have to wait until you are dying to give yourself permission to wear the kind of clothes that YOU LIKE! And to look the way you want. Do what you like. DO IT NOW!

For everyone this experience is different. For me it was wearing less tight-fitting clothes that were less restrictive. My new healthy body wanted to move more and stretch more, so loose, baggy pants and Karate Gi pants were more my new style. Since I was more active, sweats, t-shirts and more casual clothes were better and also clothes that I could layer depending on my workout and physical activity schedule. Some of my patients were just the opposite and wanted tighter clothes to show off their new healthy and fit body that they had worked so hard to make.

Once you start _singing your own song_ you end up realizing you are the coolest anyway, a trend setter. People notice your attitude and they want you.

So get out there and find some natural fiber new clothes. It's not difficult. If you can't find the types of clothes that you're used to wearing made from cotton or wool, then take the leap and experiment with a new clothing style. What we're creating here is a new healthier you, so this new you should look a little bit different. Try a few more colors than what you usually wear while you're at it.

OH YEAH, YOUR FEET

Ask any electrician, if you put your finger into a light bulb socket you will get a shock, but it won't kill you. That is because you are probably wearing sneakers and standing on some carpet or wood floor. On the other hand, if you put your finger into a light bulb socket, and you are barefooted standing outside on the dirt ground or in a water puddle, you will become a human welder. You will burn, fry and possibly die. This is because you are now GROUNDED.

Being grounded simply means that your body is now in contact with the ground and your body is now completing the electrical circuit into the ground. The electricity can now pass through you and pass out of your body and actually into the ground. _"Don't try this at home, I am a professional."_

Every second of your life your body creates electricity. This isn't some new age hocus pocus; it's medical and scientific fact. _Your body really makes electricity._ When a medical doctor hooks up electro-cardiogram pads and wires to your chest or an electroencephalogram pads and wires to your head, they are actually measuring the electricity that your heart and your brain are making, generating and sparking.

With most people in modern life, they are making lots of electricity, but it builds up and up inside their body and never gets a chance to dissipate or discharge.

The only way that this electricity, just like an electrical circuit, can discharge is for your naked body, or at least your naked feet, to be in contact with the earth.

SUN AND AIR BATHING

A hundred years ago naturopathic and medical hospitals knew the healing power of getting sun and fresh air every day, and getting outside. Going outside *naked* and getting sun over your entire body, and letting your body *air out* and getting your bare feet on the ground, these acts were well-established as important healing tools.

Well, nothing has changed and they still are today, except that most people have no place to do this and it isn't politically correct anymore. It's healing correct, though.

I used to suggest to my patients to get naked at night and get out into their backyards at least, and run and roll around. It did them a world of good. But if all else fails, get your shoes and socks off and walk barefooted, shuffling your feet in the grass or in the dirt for 15 minutes at night. This will sufficiently ground you and help discharge stored up and stagnant physical electricity.

If you can, the absolute best is to get into water. Come on, jump into the ocean, or a lake, a quarry, a puddle, squirt yourself with the garden hose or dump a pail of water over your head, GET WET! Getting wet is one of the most powerful therapies I had in my clinic. I literally used to take patients for a walk on the beach in front of my clinic, and when they would least expect it, I would throw their butt in, clothes and all, summer or winter. It was my secret weapon to cure insomnia and heal disease.

Finally, also consider just going barefoot when you can. A few years ago I decided to do a shoe fast for a month and wear nothing on my feet for 30 days. I even went to meetings in suits, in the city, to restaurants, all over and you know what happened? NOTHING, nobody even noticed, ___so let the dogs out___!

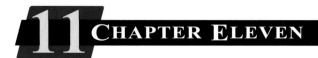

CHAPTER ELEVEN

NATURAL CLEANING

On your body and in your house, start using natural cleansing products or none at all.

WHY SHOULD I?

What you use to clean your body and your house is killing you.

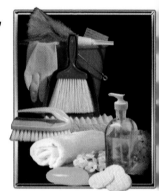

FACTS

- Over 72,000 new synthetic chemicals have been developed since WWII and less than 2% of them have been tested for Toxicity. Many are known to cause Birth Defects, Cancer and damage the Liver, Kidneys and Brain. Most have NEVER been tested for long term effects.

- The average American home has more toxic chemicals in it than a chemistry lab did in the early 1900's.

- The National Institute of Occupational Safety and Health has found over 2,500 toxic chemicals just in common cosmetics that cause cancer tumors, reproductive disease and mutate unborn children.

- A recent EPA study concluded that air inside American homes is up to 70 TIMES more polluted than outdoor air and that toxic fumes from common household cleaners cause cancer.

- Common bleach has been linked to causing breast cancer along with laundry detergents, household cleaners and pesticides. Bleach has also been linked to reproductive failure in men and behavioral problems in children.

How To Do It?

I grew up in the fabulous fifties where I never even heard of the word pollution, all drugs were wonder drugs and my mother who had supposedly grey hair (which was really bluish purple but we didn't tell her), well, her sink, dresser and night stand were covered with endless wonder beauty and personal care items. Our kitchen and laundry room in the basement was a chemical goldmine, better than most teenagers chemistry sets today, where my brother and I could make anything just short of nuclear warheads.

But in the last half century we have learned, just like we have with pharmaceutical drugs, that many of these supposedly harmless cleaners, conditioners and personal care items are extremely toxic. Some are even lethal.

Natural Products may not be perfect, but all the stuff labeled "natural" is a whole lot better than what we buy in a regular drug store. And I don't want you using any deodorants or perfumes or cologne. If you smell, you can use some pure plant essential oils, but no plant *perfume* oils. Make sure that all soaps that you wash with and everything you put on your body is natural and has no toxic chemicals in it. I mean everything from body soap, shampoos and hair conditioners, toothpaste, mouthwash, toothpicks, dental floss, moisturizing creams and lotions, EVERYTHING! And don't forget your hair dyes, hair color, lacquer, sprays, gels, dippity goo— whatever. You men, too. Those chemicals go right through the pores of your scalp and circulate into your brain. That's probably why some people's thoughts are as stiff as their hair.

And NEVER, NEVER, NEVER use anti-perspirant. Your body and skin sweating is elimination and if you stop it you are pushing poison back into your body. If you smell, and often people do for a while as they are getting healthy, cover it up with pure plant essential oils.

Look, I was born at night but not *last night*. I know that *everything* from a health food store is not always necessarily better, but it probably is. I also know that it costs more but don't let me find you being cheap with yourself when it comes to healing disease and getting healthy.

And while you're at it, get all those cans and bottles out from under your sink and take them to some toxic disposal site.

In tens of thousands of independent studies conducted all over the world, common household chemicals, from all purpose degreasers and window cleaners to common kitchen items such as plastic wrap, <u>have all been found to be a harmful, if not serious, health risk</u>.

I remember seeing a show on public television about a decade ago that showed the results of ordinary cleaning products on people who had never used them. I remember seeing primitive natives that basically lived naked and in the forest, made to put on typical clothes that we wear every day that had been laundered in typical laundry soap, and within a few hours to a few days, it burnt their skin. Many were burnt so bad they had to be hospitalized, and as I remember, a few died.

The only difference with us is that we have all been so poisoned for so many generations now our bodies have built up some resistance to this chemical onslaught. But in the last decade numerous scientific and medical studies have confirmed that many common diseases in America are negatively impacted by these products, if not directly caused by them. Cancers such as Lung Cancer, Liver Cancer, Pancreatic Cancer, Blood Cancer (Leukemia), Brain Cancer, Colon Cancer and Kidney Cancer have all been linked to toxic chemical exposure. In fact with almost all cancers today, the leading culprit is pointing towards toxic chemical exposure.

When the average person hears this they are looking to blame the local landfill, heavy industry or power plant. Although these industries can be contributors, the exposure level of toxic chemicals and gases is much higher in the average household than in the air outside the house, even in the big cities. (see the FACTS at the beginning of this chapter.)

<u>The Bottom Line:</u>
Clean yourself and your home, but don't make yourself sick with what you are using to clean up with.

DR. SCHULZE QUOTE: "Tomorrow is what you BELIEVE and DO Today!"

12 CHAPTER TWELVE

STOP TELEVISION

Stop watching television, especially the News. Turn It Off!

WHY SHOULD I?

People who watch television for more than two hours a day have a dramatic increase in just about every serious disease known to mankind. I am talking every disease from Diabetes and Arthritis to Heart Disease, Stroke and Cancer.

This is partly due to being more sedentary and not moving while snacking on junk food. It is also because you are being emotionally stimulated, but usually in a negative way.

FACTS

- 99.9999999999999999999999999% of the people in the entire world had a pretty good day today, or at least an average day today.

- Watching television news has been scientifically and medically proven to reduce the ability of your immune system to protect your body from disease.

- American researchers have found compelling new evidence that people who spend long hours in front of the television are at increased risk of Alzheimer's disease.

HOW TO DO IT?

As I said, 99.99999999999999999999999999% of the people in the entire world had a pretty good day today, or at least an average day.

But the news media searched out and found, filmed and interviewed the .0000000000000000000000000001% of men women and children that were beaten, tortured, maimed, burned, raped, robbed, assaulted, terrorized, killed, murdered, butchered, murdered their families, stung by killer bees, bit by sharks, had their homes destroyed in flood, hurricanes, tornadoes, cyclones, thunderstorms, windstorms, earthquakes, brushfires, mudslides, high surf, hailstones, and even struck by lightning, air crashes, train wrecks, massive auto and truck collisions and barges knocking down bridges trapping people to be drowned in the dark. They found the wars, the bombings, the suicide attackers, their victims and maybe even a small piece of their leftover body, the tanks, destroyers, bombers, the terrorists, their victims, the religious wars, the yelling, screaming, fighting, demonstrations, molested and raped children, car bombings, and the very sick man who lived in a one-room apartment, kept 79 cats and slowly starved them all to death, and ate a few.

And the only short interruptions to this 30 or 60 minutes of condensed and concentrated mayhem and madness is a quick sales pitch for you to eat more sugar, junk food, take more drugs, use more toxic chemicals in your house and maybe even buy a video that has the worst disasters and police shootings on it, so bad they were censored from television, but you can buy them all on one video and view them at home over and over again.

THE FINAL BLOW

When my son was 3 and we were having a rare television viewing of a Popeye cartoon, I was getting us a drink and they interrupted the broadcast to show a live action camera shot of a man who parked his car in the middle of a bridge in Los Angeles, stopping traffic in all directions. As the policed approached he pulled out a gun, so they backed off. He then pulled out a banner and placed it on the ground for the television cameras that said "My HMO F—ked Me". He then pulled out a shotgun and as he put it into his mouth all of the cameras at various angles zoomed in. He then lit himself on fire (he had previously doused himself with gasoline) and then pulled the trigger of the 12-gauge shotgun, blowing the entire back of his head off and sending his brains splattering about a city block away, all in beautiful color with digital sound. I watched very little television up to that point in my life, but that day I turned the television off, and I've never turned it back on since.

The other day I told someone that I don't watch television and that I actually turned it off years ago. The person looked absolutely shocked and then frightened, like I was some kind of alien or sicko. And then they said, "Well, you at least watch the news, don't you?" And I said, "No, I don't watch the news either." And now they could no longer hide the total look of horror on their face. In a near-panicked and shaky voice they said, "But how do you know what's going on?"

Since when is television news what's really going on. It is certainly not a reflection of what I see and hear on a daily basis. It is not reality, or at least not reality in proportion to all the people on the earth.

PROTECT YOURSELF

Protect yourself from this mind-rotting physical, emotional and spiritual violence. Make your home a temple. Make your home a sacred place. And maybe the best way to start this process is by turning your television OFF.

Now let's take it a step further. Don't bring anything into your house that is not going to promote your higher physical and emotional self. So if you're going to eat that bad food, or express bad emotions, or whatever, do it outside your home. At the same time you will also want to get some of the things out of your house that you don't need anymore and that are making you sick. This brings us to step number 13.

DR. SCHULZE
QUOTE:

"Getting well
is EASY.
It is getting sick that
takes years of constant,
dedicated hard work."

13 CHAPTER THIRTEEN

TRASHING

Healing life-threatening degenerative disease takes a serious life-changing program. *I have found that getting rid of 1/3 of your possessions is one of the most powerful healing tools I had in the clinic.*

WHY SHOULD I?

Your possessions take your attention and focus. Getting rid of 1/3 of what you own is shock therapy. It gives you 33% more focus onto healing yourself. It is a big wake-up call.

Also, EVERYONE has some possessions that are a burden instead of making their life easier, more joyful and adding to their overall well-being. These possessions instead add stress, make you sick and are killing you!

FACTS

• When someone has a degenerative disease, something they own is making them sick, is killing them. <u>I never saw an exception to this rule</u> *(see the two patient case histories on the next page).* You will also see from my patients that getting rid of what I call toxic possessions often creates an emotional purge which creates huge leaps forward in your physical healing.

HOW TO DO IT?

I used to call this "trashing" in my clinic. Bury your possessions before they bury you. You know the crap that is in your house that I am talking about. Maybe it's all that garbage that you think are priceless relics but you know they are not.

Maybe its all those broken parts stuffed in your garage that you think you might need some day, but you never will.

Let me tell you, your kids are going to curse you some day when you die and they have to deal with it and they will end up selling all of your junk for $15 in some garage sale. Save them the time, trouble and emotional heartache and at the same time do yourself a healing favor, and get rid of it all now. THROW IT AWAY!

What about that shoebox, file box or drawer full of papers that you think is so important so you can't throw them away? You think it's important and you plan on sorting through it all one day? Trust me, you will never get to it but you will stress yourself out thinking about it. Do yourself a gigantic favor. Walk the box out to the trash. Let it go. Drop it and throw it away and scream, "YAHOO, thank you Dr. Schulze!"

If you throw away one-third of all the stuff in your house, that will be a powerful healing in itself. Remember, this stuff is not you, and it distracts you from living and it will make you sick. GET RID OF IT.

HOUSE CALLS

I love house calls. Although they are now a thing of the past along with vinyl records and 8-track tapes, I still advise all practitioners reading this book to do them. They are a BIG EYE-OPENER. For me I often discovered *toxic* possessions and when we got rid of them the patients had a huge healing.

Usually I would tell each new patient that I wanted to see them for about 10 visits, one visit every other week, so their entire program would take about 20 weeks. In this period of time I would give my patients a series of natural healing projects and programs to accomplish, like my Health Building Food Program, my Bowel Detoxification Program and my 5 Day Cleansing and Detoxification Program.

By the end of 10 visits or 20 weeks my patients would be feeling better than they had in years, if not their entire life. And of course, almost always their disease and illness would be gone.

But whenever a patient had a degenerative disease or a life-threatening illness, I would often need more than 10 office visits. I also wanted to get to know them better and get more *personal* with them. Just like any great detective I needed more facts, even so-called trivial ones, to *crack the case.* So I would make the 3rd or 4th visit a *house call* and go to the patients home instead of them coming to me.

Often my patients would think this is a bit strange because it just isn't done these days, but I would make it very clear to them, my house call wasn't an option, it was a necessity.

When I would get to their house I would tell the patient that I wanted the full tour, no room left out. I could see them getting nervous already. I would often like to start with the living room and the bedroom and bathroom. After all, I already knew that they had thrown out all of their junk food to make a good impression so I wasn't going to go to the kitchen until later.

I am very good at what I do, I am a GREAT detective, so usually within the first 10 minutes I would find it, a possession so toxic that it was killing them.

COLITIS CURED INSTANTLY

I was seeing a young patient in her apartment. She was 19 or 20 and had colitis so bad that she hadn't been to work in several days. Her employer was worried so I checked in on her as a favor to her employer. She was not a patient of mine but knew of me and was expecting me. She had constant diarrhea-like bowel movements, about 20 a day, and was very sick.

We talked for just a minute and I noticed hanging in an *unusually* prominent place in the middle of her empty bedroom wall was her college graduation diploma. She had graduated with honors at the very top of her class, something many people are proud of. When I remarked about it I could immediately see that her whole body language changed. I asked her more and she began to get sick.

As it turned out she told me she absolutely hated college, every minute, every hour, every day, every week, every month and every one of her years. It turned out that her parents said that they would not continue to support her, they would shut their financial support off, if she didn't go to college. She saw no choice. She went and hated every minute of it, yet she placed her diploma on the most prominent place in the whole room.

I asked her if I could see it closer. She looked a bit nervous but said yes so I took it down off the wall for closer inspection. I then asked her if I could look at it even closer and actually take it out of the glass fronted frame. She said no but I explained to her that if I was going to be able to help her that I had to look at everything very closely. I think she thought that I was looking for some rare fungus or Legionnaire's Disease, and, looking very nervous but with a shaky voice, she said OK, take it out.

When I slipped her college magna cum laud diploma out of the frame I knew that I had struck gold. She started to tense up all over. Tears started running down her cheeks and she started to cry and babble. **I love babble; that is when some of the most important information comes out.** She was actually having some dialogue with her parents like I told you how much I hated college and you would never listen and made me go. She lost the sense that I was even in the room and I said hey look, and with her diploma in my hands I tore it right in half.

Well, I got more physical shock out of her body than if I would have double tapped her with a 44 caliber magnum. WOW, she flew back flat on to the bed at first and then immediately shot forward just like the film of JFK when he was shot in Dallas. She immediately clutched her abdomen in pain, looked up at me sobbing and gasping just to see me rip the halves in half again. She vomited.

The long and short of this patient and her colitis is that with a food program change, some Intestinal Formula #2 and a few days, her colitis was gone and never returned. I had found her colitis irritant. A daily reminder of the worst years of her life and her parents abandonment. I got rid of it and she healed herself.

BREAST CANCER CURED

I had a patient with a malignant breast tumor. It was her first bout with cancer but it was killing her. During her house call, as she was walking me down the hall after I saw her bedroom, there was a locked door. I asked her to open it and she said, oh no, I haven't opened that room in years. All the more reason to open it, I thought, and asked her to get the key. She did it reluctantly, so I knew I was on to something.

When I finally got her to open the door it was like a children's museum frozen in time, spooky, children's furniture, toys, games, everything. Much of it was covered up with sheets. I asked her to explain and she told me that it was her daughter's room who had died as a child a few years previous. I believe the child was about 8. I could see when I was in the room that it was extremely painful for her to be in the room with me.

I have heard people say that a parent should never outlive their children and being a parent I can totally understand this logic. A parent is never prepared to deal with their child's death. But I could see that this room was, to her, her unburied child, a tomb, and she had to walk by it many times every day, and I can imagine what grief, anger, sadness and hell went through her mind *and body* every time she walked by it. And I knew that it had to go.

We sat down and I told her this room must be dismantled, opened up, cleaned out and turned into something new. She asked me what she should do with all of her daughter's possessions and I said she needed to throw them away. She started crying and looked at me like I was insane. A woman's breasts are all about nurturing so in that moment I not only knew that she had to throw all of this away, she had to do it NOW, and I told her so.

I was quite convincing. After all it was a matter of life or death. I made her carry and drag everything herself out to the backyard to a big trash dumpster. What a sight. Sobbing hysterically, snot running out of her nose, drooling, gagging. On the second load she had an incredible very sharp pain in her breast and doubled over. She said it was the worst pain she had in that breast ever. I told her to continue and it took most of the day. At one point she collapsed in the driveway and scraped both of her knees bloody and I just let her lay there and cry. I've said it before: *sympathy is between shit and syphilis in the dictionary and I NEVER saw it help anyone, EVER, to heal themselves.*

I am not a total sadistic bastard but I did let her writhe in her experience. I didn't want to lessen anything. In fact, I was there to keep it going and prod her along.

Well, the long and short of this is that it turned out to be the absolute turning point for this woman. She went on to bury her daughter emotionally and also to heal her breast cancer. I have talked to her from time to time and she gets better with age and has never had the cancer return.

Note: my patient case histories often revealed that people who develop cancer almost always have some horrible experience in the previous two years before the cancer surfaced, an experience they could not deal with.

The Bottom Line...

Trashing, getting rid of accumulated toxic waste in your life, is as healing as getting rid of toxic waste in your body.

14 CHAPTER FOURTEEN

RELAXATION

Now that I have told you what to drink, eat, how to move, breathe, cleanse, and what to wear...now I want you to do NOTHING.

WHY SHOULD I?

The results are in: regular relaxation reduces stress, protects your health, helps you heal disease and increases your longevity . . . . so take a break.

FACTS

- In America and most modern, civilized countries, STRESS has been proven by many medical researchers to be the #1 cause of vitality loss, health deterioration, illness, disease, premature aging and even death.

- The famous vegetarian cardiologist Dr. Dean Ornish completed a study that shocked the medical world, proving that his patients could not only stop the progression of coronary artery blockage and disease with lifestyle changes, but that they could actually reverse the disease and clear their blocked arteries on his program, without drugs and surgery. His program basically consisted of a vegetarian food program, about an hour of aerobic exercise a day, some stretching and 30 minutes of stress reduction relaxation every day. An additional enlightening fact discovered during his research was that many people followed almost the whole program, the vegetarian food, the exercise, the stretching, almost everything, except that they just skipped the 30-minute <u>relaxation</u> stress reduction part, <u>and they did not get well</u>! The research results proved that relaxation was a fundamental key aspect of his program that determined the patients' success or failure.

- **It is estimated that at least one-third (or 16.6 million) of the 50 million Americans who have been diagnosed with Hypertension (High Blood Pressure) and are using anti-hypertensive drugs prescribed from their medical doctor actually do NOT have a physical cause for their disease, like constricted or blocked arteries, high cholesterol, diabetes, etc. The cause of their disease is simply heightened levels of stress.**

HOW TO DO IT?

In the first years of my Martial Arts study, when I was just a teenager, I was in a very traditional Japanese school. My parents were both dead and I was a very angry kid and my *Sensei* (teacher) was a very enlightened man and recognized this. Therefore he demanded that if I wanted his instruction, then I must attend meditation classes at a Zen Buddhist monastery at least 3 times a week for 5 years or he wouldn't teach me. He also made me sweep the floor and clean out the *dojo* (practice hall) for my entire first year at his school.

At the monastery I was taught *zazen* or Zen meditation, which was simply the art of sitting very still, quieting your breath and quieting your mind, until your body and mind go silent. It took me TWO ENTIRE YEARS before I experienced my first *satori,* or quieting of my mind, and the bliss and healing that swells from this experience. Most Americans (in fact, most people in the world) have never experienced this physical and emotional shutdown and bliss.

<u>What is my point?</u> Well, I don't expect anyone reading this book to do what I did, but trust me, most people have no idea of what true and total relaxation is.

<u>Years later in my clinic</u> I saw many patients who had unbelievable levels of stress and it was literally killing them. They had tried to take chemical drugs to lessen the diseases that were the after and side effects of their stress but it didn't help. I saw everything from Hypertension *High Blood Pressure,* Cardiac Arrhythmia and Tachycardia or *Irregular or Speeded Up Heart Beat,* Angina Pectoris or *Heart Pain,* Stroke, Nervous Disorders from nervous ticks, Depression, Insomnia to full blown

Neurological Diseases and Nervous Breakdowns, Immune Failure, and Cancer. I have seen almost every disease known brought on by the body first being weakened from STRESS.

To avoid taking a break these patients had done everything from taking every sedative and anti-depressive drug known to acupuncture and feng suei, but there is no substitute for relaxation. They had literally done everything, except of course DOING NOTHING.

So I would demand that these patients take a few weeks, if not a month, off work and I was shocked that when they returned from their vacation, THEY NEEDED A VACATION FROM THEIR VACATION! They were typical Americans, you know, see 27 cities in 5 days. Even if they stayed stationary on their vacation they played golf, tennis, water sports, went out dancing at night or, worse, watched television for hours. MOST PEOPLE DON'T HAVE THE FAINTEST IDEA OF HOW TO DO NOTHING, ABSOLUTELY NOTHING!

When I say RELAX I mean DOING NOTHING! I mean sitting, better yet lying, down in the grass, woods, beach, backyard, bedroom, preferably wherever there aren't other people nearby, breathing, letting your body relax and drift away. At first many people will fall asleep; that's OK. That is just your body asking for more rest after years of coffee and their hyper-adrenal-whipped and stimulated life. After practicing this type of relaxation for a while you often won't fall asleep but will fall into a deep state of relaxation.

This deep relaxation is one of the most healing things you can do for your body, mind and spirit. It is pure and absolute rest. You are shutting the system down completely except your minimal life support systems. This rest will recharge your system and give your body the space to heal disease. After all, any machine that is left running constantly will burn out and break down. The human body is not a 16-hour continuous duty machine.

In the clinic I have seen the addition of daily rest periods into peoples' lives heal disease and create healing miracles.

Often the best way to begin is to cut your lunch hour in half and spend the second half of your lunchtime to relax. Even if you can only have 15 minutes, even 5 minutes of quite time every day, this can add years to your life.

I had one high stress executive that literally couldn't get a minute's rest at his 16-hour a day job. Even when he tried to just take a few minutes quiet at his desk he would almost always be interrupted. So I instructed him, as well as many other patients, to go into the bathroom, sit on the toilet leaving the toilet seat down, turn out the lights, spray a little air essential oils, close their eyes, breathe deep, and disappear for 5 to 10 minutes. Because the toilet is often the only place where people will leave you alone.

Many of my patients later told me that this *toilet meditation* practice literally *saved their life!*

MORE MEDICAL CARE MAY KILL US QUICKER

In America we spend more money per person, more than any other country in the world, on medical care. We *supposedly* have the brightest scientific minds, the best medical technology and equipment, the finest hospitals, the most in-depth research, the most powerful drugs, and yet ironically Americans don't even make it into the top 20 countries with the longest life spans. **This proves without a doubt that we can't buy our health and longevity with doctors, drugs and hospitals, but that we must *earn* our health**.

Many of the countries where the people outlive Americans like Australia, France, Sweden, Spain, Italy, Greece, Canada, The Netherlands, Norway, Belgium, Austria, Luxembourg, Iceland, Finland and Israel are considered mostly rural, backward and supposedly uncivilized or *third world* countries that have poorer medical care than America. Many of these people have NO MEDICAL CARE AT ALL, EVER! This is a very embarrassing fact that partially reflects that our **American over-aggressive use of medical intervention, surgery and drugs may actually shorten, not lengthen, our lives** (how embarrassing for the biggest industry in America).

Other researchers are saying it's because the French drink more red wine or the Italians eat more Garlic and are frantically looking for something in their water or food that might be this rare chemical *fountain of youth.*

Meanwhile, any idiot visiting these countries can quickly see their increased longevity is not only due to their reduced medical care but also their reduced level of stress (or none at all).

(see next page)

LESSONS I LEARNED FROM TEACHING AROUND THE WORLD

SPAIN

Many years ago I was teaching a course on Natural Healing and Herbal Medicine in a small town in the southern coastal area of Spain. I was staying in a room on the roof of a building off a small road at the end of town. The roads just a few miles inland from the Mediterranean Sea in the coast of Spain, France, Monaco and even Italy are often very mountainous with twisting and turning roads with steep cliffs and drop-offs.

This town was a coastal mountain village way up in the hills with a very high bridge in the middle of town. In the evening I saw a huge crowd at this bridge; I think everyone in town was there. I watched and figured that someone had fallen off the bridge, or jumped off, or a car had gone over the side. After about an hour I couldn't stand my curiosity any more and ran over to the bridge to see what all the commotion was about and why this crowd had gathered, what had happened.

All that was happening was that they were talking and laughing with their friends and neighbors and discussing the day's events and the elders were telling stories, a nightly event in many small towns across the world. I didn't recognize this because we don't do it anymore and this is one of the reasons that we die sooner than they do.

ENGLAND

When I was teaching a course in England I was staying in a castle a few miles outside a small town. I needed to make a telephone call and couldn't get the one telephone in the building to work. I remembered seeing a gatekeeper's house at the entry to the castle where it looked like someone lived so I wandered down there in hopes of making my phone call.

I knocked on the door about 10 a.m. and as a very old woman opened the door I was immediately hit with a wave of the very strong, horrible smell of urine. As I was holding my nose I realized this smell was originating from a frying pan where she was frying two large cow kidneys on her stove. She was also smoking a cigarette and in the other hand had a glass of sherry. Drinking, smoking and eating organ meats all at 10 a.m. in the morning!

I couldn't help myself and asked her how old she was, secretly hoping she was only 25 and that her degenerated lifestyle had severely aged her prematurely, but I was wrong. She was exactly 100 years old, born in 1884. Well here she is, smoking, drinking and frying organ meat all before noon and alive and well at 100. Her cholesterol level in her blood was so elevated for so many years that I could see her *coronary arcus, an iris marking reflecting chronic elevated cholesterol levels,* from six feet away. Sure there are *George Burns* genetic exceptions to the fundamentals of good healthy living, or was my career about to end?

I asked her if I could use her telephone and she belly-laughed in her coarse and gravelly voice and said, "I haven't ever had a telephone." I said to her, but what if you need to talk to someone, and she said, "I need to talk to people every day, so I just walk into town (6 miles roundtrip EXERCISE) and have a chat with my friends (RELAXATION).

I spent a good part of the day chatting with this amazing woman and realized, sure, genetics has plenty to do with longevity, but it was obvious that this woman's 100 years of the most decadent and health-destroying lifestyle was offset not only by her powerful genetic constitution but also her daily exercise, RELAXATION and having virtually NO STRESS!

FRANCE

I have an acquaintance who is one of the most powerful attorneys in France and while in Paris I was staying at his house. The first day I was there I came home for lunch about two in the afternoon and the housekeeper informed me that he was in bed and had been there for over an hour. I went in and said, "Oh my God, what's wrong?" and he looked at me very surprised and said, "I don't know, what's wrong?" and I said, "Well you are in bed in the middle of the afternoon," and he said, "I rest in bed every day after my lunch." Here one of the most high-powered attorneys in Paris walks home every day for his 1 hour lunch and then takes a 1 to 2 hour rest or nap in bed and then walks back to work for his afternoon work session. And we say it's some secret ingredient in the French Red Wine that gives them less heart attacks and makes them live longer.

ITALY

I was teaching a course in Italy to middle-aged medical doctors and nurses and there was one student in the class that kept interrupting me. He was pretending to ask questions but was actually making statements. I guess he wanted to be the teacher. Finally another frustrated student in the room stood up and said, "Hey, why don't you just shut up, we all came here to see and hear Dr. Schulze, NOT YOU!, but you keep talking and talking and talking and interrupting and we aren't getting to hear Dr. Schulze, so just shut your mouth."

The talking student shut up but I was embarrassed and frightened. I thought that maybe they would physically fight. Heck, in America I have seen lawsuits for slander and assault for less being said.

So I figured the best thing to do was to call an early break so the students could cool off, settle down and lighten up. When I walked out into the hallway I was shocked at what I saw. These two same men were talking and one of them even had his arm around the other. They weren't mad, angry, or hostile. I have now come to learn that in many countries it is not considered rude to express yourself even if it is done in a bit of a harsh manner. I have learned that many people blow off and VENT their steam, say what's on their mind, they are honest, and nobody seems to make a big deal about it. I was brought up to hold it in until you either get sick, have a heart attack, grow a cancer tumor or commit murder.

I discovered that the only person who was stressed out about this situation was ME. Since then I have learned to be more Italian. Sure, the Garlic may have something to do with why they can eat so much meat and still have very low cholesterol levels, less heart attacks and strokes, but their *Relaxed attitude* is what keeps them living longer.

P.S. I have spent some time over the last three summers in the Tuscany area of Italy where I am remodeling a very old farmhouse. I like the area because the fall weather is warm and similar to Southern California where I live most of the year, and it is great Echinacea growing country, but that is where the similarity stops.

The one very obvious difference is that the pace of work, and life in general, is much, much slower (as it is in most countries outside the United States). I figure at the current rate of work being done it will take about another 147 years to finish the house.

Unlike in America, talking, eating, breaks, socializing, getting sidetracked, getting lost, taking a few days off, or a week or a month, picking mushrooms, going fishing or hunting, taking the dog for a walk and even getting drunk all seem to be just as important as building a house and making money.

Although I prefer a faster pace I am slowly learning the Italian art of moving a bit slower and relaxing more. Maybe it is better to have a little less but to be able to enjoy life a little longer. My house might take longer to build at this pace, but the pace will help me to stay alive so I will be around a lot longer to enjoy it more.

15 CHAPTER FIFTEEN

EXPRESS YOURSELF

Unexpressed emotions, whether positive or negative, make you sick. You must learn to express them, EXPRESS YOURSELF, and get them out!

WHY SHOULD I?

Part of expressing yourself is letting it out—your thoughts, your feelings, your emotions, your anger, your rage, your love. Whatever is brewing up inside of you, it's healthy to get it out.

Unexpressed emotions build up inside you, inside your brain. That is why you can remember them. They also build up inside your heart and soul. Let it go.

Being emotionally constipated is as deadly as being physically constipated in your colon.

FACTS

* Besides Type A and Type B personalities, medical doctors are now creating a new Type C personality. The Type C personality is now defined and characterized by the type of person who holds it all in. A person who no matter how much stress they are feeling, they don't show it. Doctors now refer to this Type C personality as the CANCER TYPE. This is simply because this type of personality is extremely common in people who develop cancer.

* Tears have been found to contain many metabolic chemicals from your body, especially ones that build up during stress. Tears are no longer thought to be just a byproduct of strong emotion but are now known to be part of a chemical release, a stress release.

HOW TO DO IT?

We already talked about getting rid of waste, toxins, poisons and increasing your elimination. This is the same thing. You might just call it emotional waste or emotional toxins, so let's call this process EMOTIONAL ELIMINATION, but in any case you've got to get it out.

Trust me, you don't want to hold on to this stuff.

Emotional poisons will grow a tumor just as fast as chemical poisons.

Don't hold on to them and grow a tumor. Don't hold them in and create a disease. Let it out; scream it out if necessary, you can always ask for forgiveness later. But whatever you do, get it out.

This is as important as getting out toxic bowel or liver waste. Unexpressed emotions, even love, can make you sick if you don't learn to express them and get them out. Express who you are.

I totally understand that this doesn't come easy for most people. This is simply because most of us were taught and brought up to SUPPRESS our emotions. Stuff it, Stifle it, Bury it, and just shut up and take it. This made us all sick.

Once you get the hang of it, it gets easier and easier. I find that people LOVE the truth, they love straight talk, they welcome it because it is so rare. My powerful honesty and saying it as I see it, well, a lot of people love me for being so open. Sure, there are always a few who write letters telling me to burn in hell, but come on, there are always a few people like that. I always say that everyone is entitled to their own *wrong* opinion. We all need to lighten it up a few notches and let it out.

Expressing what is on your mind is a POWERFUL HEALING TOOL. I had many patients with throat cancer, thyroid disease, lung diseases like asthma, emphysema, bronchitis, allergies, even lung cancer, brain diseases, nerve diseases and heart diseases from hypertension to cardiac arrhythmia . . . . make huge leaps in their healing process by learning to express themselves and getting all of that built up emotion OUT!

Many of them noticed a big physical healing moment, sometimes a total cure, from just expressing something that they had been holding on to for years.

GETTING IT OFF
THEIR CHEST

Getting it off of my chest literally helped me heal my deformed heart. Sometimes I think my heart was deformed simply because I was *crushed* by my parents dying but I never told anyone that. <u>I crushed myself and couldn't get it off my chest. Sounds like a recipe for heart disease, doesn't it</u>? That helped my street survival outside, but was killing me *inside*.

In order for me to heal my heart disease I also learned to express positive affirmations WITH GUSTO! It is fun. I only bowl once a year at our company bowling tournament. So since I don't get any practice, when I bowl I say, "Hey, I'm a great bowler." Because of my positive affirmation I bowl better and I have more fun bowling. Sure I could focus on a gutter ball or two but all I remember is the four strikes I had in a row last year, which is because I AM A GREAT BOWLER!

So express yourself AND USE YOUR POSITIVE AFFIRMATIONS TOO. Speak up. Say who you are and you'll be able to live out your dreams instead of living your nightmares.

TRY IT
I Love Myself!
I Love My Life!
YAHOO!

When you see yourself in the mirror tomorrow morning I want to hear you scream YES, WHAT A HUNK! . . . . all the way to my house in Malibu, California.

DR. SCHULZE

QUOTE:

"Trust yourself, trust your inner voice, and stop asking so many questions.

Quiet yourself, don't panic, and all of the right answers will come at the right time."

170 COMMON SENSE HEALTH AND HEALING

16 CHAPTER SIXTEEN

HELP OTHERS

Help someone every day.

WHY SHOULD I?

While everyone else is rushing around, I want you to stop and take the time to help someone. It's fun, you'll feel good and it is healing to your body, mind and spirit.

FACTS

- Beyond the good Christian "Do Unto Others" or the Buddhists and Hindu "Good Karma", over the years numerous physiological and psychological tests have been done regarding people who take the time to help other people, the so-called Good Samaritan, and those that don't. The test and study results are always obviously positive for those that stop and help others. What scientists have referred to as the Good Samaritan effect has been shown to be beneficial to heart disease, neurological diseases, even cancer and a host of emotional disorders from stress-related diseases to depression and anxiety.

- For many of my patients it created a moment in time that shifted their attention from constantly dwelling on themselves and their disease to something and someone else. This proved to be a very healing and magical moment.

HOW TO DO IT?

The other day I was driving home and there was a man stuck in the middle of the road. His pickup truck had died and he was marooned in the middle lane of Pacific Coast Highway during the worst, *Friday rush hour traffic*. People were blowing their horns and they were screaming at him. One woman even drove by and threw him the finger and I swear, after she passed I saw the bumper sticker on her car which read "Imagine World Peace". Well, honey, world peace starts with you, with action, not your imagination. Maybe she was driving someone else's car.

So I put on my emergency flashers and actually parked behind this man and very carefully walked out into congestion of stop and go cars with pissed off drivers like an angry mob behind the steering wheels of cars. I walked up to him and asked what I could do to help him. He said, "Please, can you help get me get out of here?" The poor man was terrified that these people almost wanted him dead. So the only thing I could figure out was to push his car with mine.

Now I had just gotten my new car a few weeks earlier, and when I was pushing him a passing motorist even yelled to me that I was scraping my bumper. Guys, it's only a bumper. Plastic, metal, whatever. I get as attached to my toys as much as the next person, but <u>this was an incredible opportunity to help someone.</u> I may never get this chance again and I want my healing moment. So yes, I did scratch my bumper. But now whenever I see that scratch it's a wonderful reminder to me to help other people every day.

Look for them. Seek them out. Hey, they're out there. It's up to you to find them. I found the secret to seeing them. All you have to do is slow down a little bit, breathe, quiet yourself, stop talking and look around. Get out of your head a bit, and all of a sudden they appear like magic.

Someone that needs your help.

17 CHAPTER SEVENTEEN

LAUGH MORE

I want you to learn 1,000 jokes, only kidding,
<u>*NO I AM NOT KIDDING*</u>*!*

WHY SHOULD I?

Being sincere is good, but being too serious is not. Stress damages your immune ability and numerous medical studies have found that stress is the preliminary cause of most disease. Stress Kills! A good laugh a day literally keeps the doctor away.

FACTS

- It only takes a few muscles to smile, but about five times more to frown. This shows that it uses more energy and depletes your vitality to be upset.

- There are hundreds of metabolic shifts and changes that take place in the human body when you laugh. I could bore you with the science, but come on friends, that's too serious, because YOU CAN FEEL YOURSELF CHANGE WHEN YOU LAUGH! IT FEELS GOOD! **<u>AND IF IT FEELS GOOD IT'S GOOD FOR YOU</u>!** Laughing relieves the stress that can kill you. It also increases almost every known aspect of your immune system. There are many reports of people who laughed their way to health actually curing Cancer, AIDS, Heart Disease and many other killer diseases, just by laughing.

- On the other hand, there are hundreds of metabolic shifts and changes in your body when you are agitated, angry and upset. YOU CAN FEEL THESE TOO and I don't have to tell you how bad they feel. And if they feel that bad they are hurting you. It's that simple. Negative emotions are killers and getting healthy is about stopping killing yourself. The same way that you can laugh your way into healing disease you can upset yourself into creating disease.

HOW TO DO IT?

I want you to laugh. I mean really laugh, from deep down inside. Laugh until you cry, until snot dribbles out your nose, laugh until you pee your pants or are in so much pain your ribs hurt and you can't breathe. Actually try to die laughing.

In my clinic I would have humor night. All of my patients were invited, but my sickest patients had to attend, or I would fire them. Every week part of their program, just as important as their food program or their cleansing program, was to learn new jokes. Some had to buy joke books. We would all take our turn at stand-up comedy. Occasionally we would go out to comedy clubs and get a professional healing.

I would make my seriously ill patients learn 1,000 jokes. It was an important step in their healing. I would ask them to keep a journal of them and to get this journal out and read it every day and also recite out of it to others. Their job was to memorize the jokes and be able to tell them to perfect strangers from memory. How many jokes do you know? I had one patient that was very ill with colitis. She had 10, maybe 12 diarrhea-type hot loose stools in a day. Did you know that this type of diarrhea is actually genetic, because it runs in your jeans . . . . . Get it, runs in your jeans.

Do you know what is similar between the USS Enterprise Starship on the movie Star Trek and a roll of toilet paper. They are both designed to wipe out Klingons around Uranus.

OK, so I am guilty for having the vast majority of my jokes about chapter #5, Bowel Cleansing, but they're still jokes.

We all take ourselves and our lives way too seriously. So lighten up a little bit, in fact A LOT. Laugh more. Laughter can be more healing than fresh juice.

Start laughing today, even if you have to force it at first. Try it. Actually get hysterical. It might take some practice, especially if you've had years of training being so serious, and being in control and being cool. Years of practice being dead.

18 CHAPTER EIGHTEEN

MORE SEX

There is nothing more important than SEX because without it there is no life at all.

WHY SHOULD I?

A recent study at Scotland's Royal Edinburgh Hospital concluded that **more SEX** slows the aging process.

FACTS

- Over **10 MILLION** American women are infertile. **9 MILLION** of them used medical infertility services, spending over 2 billion dollars. Medical infertility services have an 87% failure rate.

- **500,000** American women will have their ovaries and uterus cut out this year.

- Over **60% of men** in their forties have Prostate disease and **15 MILLION** men have Prostate tumors.

- **50% of all men** have some degree of erectile dysfunction and impotence.

- The American male's sperm count has dropped to **HALF** of what it was only 70 years ago.

- Viagra sales top **2 BILLION** dollars in spite of dangerous, even lethal side effects.

- **10%** of American men can't ever get an erection.

HOW TO DO IT?

We wouldn't be here without sex. So let's have it longer and more often. Oh yeah, I know in this age of AIDS sex has become a dirty word. It's not cool to have sex anymore. We've got to be non-sexual. We shouldn't need it, shouldn't desire it. From perfume manufacturers to clothing designers to hair stylists, they're all trying to create men and women who look and smell alike and probably don't want sex anymore. Hey, orthodox religion rarely talks about sex. Usually when it does it says not to do it. Some religions even tell us to cut the tips of our penises off. Others say to remove the clitoris. This is really crazy. Is sex really uncool, unclean, unorthodox, unreligious, and unnatural? No. Hey, guys, do I have to tell you? Sex is fun. It's healthy. I don't know about you, but for me it feels pretty good and I know that God made it feel this good so that we'd do it more. So have more of it today. All of my patients regretted not having more sex in their final hours. So learn from them and have more sex now while you still can.

Potency and Fertility *is all about Survival of the Fittest*

Whether you want to believe it or not, it exists. Whether you want to believe it to be God's Divine plan, Nature's perfection or just the unfair treatment of the weak, it doesn't matter. Because every day, every second on this planet, **Natural Selection** is taking place. The fundamental process of **Survival of the Fittest** is the reality, whether you like it or not. From every cell in your body, to the corn fields of Iowa, to the jungles of Africa, the healthy and strong are winning, and the weak are losing, and dying.

Simply put, this process is the weeding out of the weak and diseased and the proliferation of the strong. Terminating the life of the weak and diseased and/or ending their ability to reproduce, and promoting the life, future and reproductive ability of the strong, naturally.

The laws of Nature are very simple, yet firm. Nature doesn't want to create sickly weak children any more than it wants weak strains of corn to prosper. This natural selection is Nature's way of guaranteeing and promoting stronger and healthier future generations. It wants the strong to survive and the weak not to be born, and if by chance the weak are born, then to be *recycled* early.

So why is it that while we are all doing our best to honor the unwell, it seems that God and Nature are still being so cruel and have turned their backs on the unfortunate? The fact is that God and Nature have always promoted that you "Reap what you Sow", (so stop blaming and quit whining) and that "Help comes to those that help themselves", (in other words, take Responsibility). Because in Nature, if you snooze, you lose, you can't reproduce, and you die.

One of the simplest ways to observe this is with plants. Weak plants get blown over by the wind, get beaten down by the rain, and get eaten up by the bugs. They grow little seed that is genetically weak and within a few seasons, GONE, forever. On the contrary, strong plants thrive, survive, adapt, produce seed and get even stronger next year. Garlic, one of our most powerful herbs on the planet, is thought to have been one of the weakest at one time. Many scientists believe that the reason it is so potently packed with anti-bacterial, anti-viral, anti-fungal and numerous other powerful protecting chemicals was because it was so attacked in the past. It learned how to adapt, grew strong and thrived while other plants withered and died.

It is the same in the animal kingdom too. Weak, diseased animals produce weaker, more-diseased offspring. Eventually these very weak animals, even if they don't get eaten, lose their ability to reproduce. It is the same for the human race.

Impotency and Infertility: Is it just bad luck or is it bad living?

Men and Women, not unlike plants and animals, as they live life in an unhealthy way, get sick and produce weaker, sickly children. When these children grow up, they often continue to live unhealthy lives, which promotes further weakness and disease. Eventually these children give birth to sick or deformed children, or stillborn children, or they abort fetuses and miscarry, or even become sterile, losing their ability to reproduce.

As we have learned, the primary functions of the human body are to repair, survive and reproduce. If your health level falls below a certain minimal point, you lose these basic functions. Earlier while writing about osteoporosis, I explained that your body is often forced to make choices for you. Well, when you are unhealthy, especially a woman, your body will always choose to protect and save you so sterility/infertility is a protective measure that your body takes, knowing that in your unhealthy state you may not be able to survive a pregnancy.

Infertility and impotency in women and men is simply a sign of poor health. If you correct the underlying causes of the poor health, you will become fertile.

Medical Doctors: are they Miracle Workers or the Anti-Christ?

The instance of Impotency and Infertility has reached epidemic proportions in America. Millions of Men and Women are sterile and as usual medical doctors have stepped up to the plate and turned unhealthy living and reproductive ignorance into a multi-billion dollar industry.

Are Medical doctors teaching sterile parents how to take responsibility for their health and live healthy lives to become fertile again? Of course not. Armed with fertility drugs, tube drills and laser beams for just ten or twenty thousands dollars, medical doctors will try to FORCE your body to do something that God and Nature have denied.

To clarify the issue, just because I am using the terms Anti-Christ, God and Nature in the above statement, THIS IS NOT A RELIGIOUS OR MORAL DEBATE! On the contrary, it is simply a scientific one. The bottom line is that your body is protecting you and does not want you to be able to have children and there are very good and very natural reasons for this.

<u>FOR MEN,</u> it is simple. When you are weak, toxic and sick your sperm count goes down. Today, due to modern living, American males have half the sperm count they had 70 years ago. Also when you are unhealthy your hormone levels go down, your circulation gets clogged and you can even lose your ability to get an erect penis. Nature's response to sickness and disease is the loss of your reproductive ability because Nature resists and sometimes refuses to allow the procreation of sickness and disease. I know, some of you men out there are thinking that you are reasonably healthy. Well, think again. Nowadays what most people think of as good health I consider a state of managed disease. Losing your ability to procreate, your potency, is a grave sign of bad health.

FOR WOMEN it is twofold. The above that applies for Men also applies to you. When you are weak, toxic and sick your hormone levels become imbalanced. You may stop ovulating, which basically means no release of eggs for fertilization. Even if you ovulate, your uterus may be toxic and infected and may not be able to hold or feed the fetus.

Also when you are weak, sick, diseased, unhealthy, obese, anorexic, stressed out, crazy, whatever, **a woman's body has a perfect natural safety/survival mechanism that PROTECTS YOU.** Your body knows that you are ill, and that any more physical or emotional stress (like carrying a child for nine months) could kill you. One of the most basic functions of the human body is survival, so temporary sterilization is your body's way of protecting you from killing yourself. If a woman does get pregnant, and at the same time gets sicker, often the woman spontaneously aborts the fetus. This again is not a curse but a blessing. Your body knew that your life would be in danger if you went to full term so it aborts the unborn child in order to save you. It may also be that your lack of health caused defects in the fetus and again this is Nature's way of weeding out the sick and weak. Would you rather have a deformed, sick and dying child? Would you rather be dead?

If God and Nature are saying NO, then YOU have to say YES!

If you can't have children, then it is time to get to work. In the clinic I had thousands of couples that were told by every type of Obstetrician, Gynecologist and Reproductive Specialist that they could never have any babies without powerful drugs, surgery and expensive laboratory procedures. How dare they! How dare these Godless butchers claim to foresee the future.

In my clinic what I experienced is that EVERY couple that wanted children, EVERY ONE OF THEM HAD BABIES. That's right, every couple, no matter what scientific horror stories they were told by their medical doctors-- **No matter how many Miscarriages, No matter how many Abortions, No matter how much Scar Tissue, No matter how long it had been since the last Menstrual Cycle, No matter how bad their Hormones were Imbalanced**-- were able to have children if they were willing to get healthy. I learned never to underestimate the power of Natural Healing and getting healthy when it comes to everything from sperm counts and impotency to ovulation and infertility.

Always remember, God and Nature both want you to have children. There is nothing more important, because without the ability to procreate, there would be no life at all. All you need to do is get healthy.

19 CHAPTER NINETEEN

LISTEN TO YOURSELF

Create some quiet time every day. Some time to breathe, to meditate and to practice listening to your inner voice.

WHY SHOULD I?

There is much more to life here on earth than what you can see and what you can actually touch and put your finger on. I always talk about what you feel in your guts, in your heart, in your soul, and about following the voice of God that is within you, that is within all of us. So have some quiet time every day. Some time to breathe, to meditate, *AND LISTEN* . . . .

FACTS

- After 20 years of clinical practice, interviewing thousands of people and helping them to heal every disease known, I can tell you one thing that I know for sure is **A FACT!**

  If you feel it in your heart, If you feel it in your guts, If you feel it in your soul,

  Whatever you feel, **IT'S RIGHT, 100% OF THE TIME!**

HOW TO DO IT?

If you don't know how, and you can't hear yourself anymore, that's OK. We have spent generations and our whole life numbing, squashing, ignoring and silencing our inner voice.

The public school system and my so-called *education* did its best job to kill my daydreaming, my imagination, my free thinking, my intuition and ingrained in me to trust knowledge, trust science, trust my teachers, *but not myself and my own feelings.*

It has taken me many years of practice to begin to hear my inner voice again. It just started *popping up* when I would be interviewing patients. I would get feelings, I would get messages. At first I tried to quiet them, I almost felt embarrassed. But they kept coming, louder and clearer and one day I listened and then more messages came. And they were ALWAYS right.

Be patient. The next time you are wondering about something or need an answer, quiet yourself, breathe, close your eyes, give yourself a moment, **and you will find that the answer was there all along,** *you just stopped listening a long time ago.*

20 CHAPTER TWENTY

LOVE LIFE

***Be bold, take the leap, shout out loud:
I LOVE MYSELF!
It all starts right here, RIGHT NOW!***

WHY SHOULD I?

If you walk around all day long frowning, not loving what you do and not loving yourself, then prepare yourself because disease and illness are not far away.

My suggestion: make up some of your own positive affirmations about how much you love yourself, how much you love your life, how much you love where you live, and how much you love your family. You love everybody and everything. Tell yourself how good you are at doing things, and the next thing you know you'll be living in love and your disease and illness will be gone.

FACTS

- It is now medically and scientifically proven that your immune cells monitor and react to your emotional dialogue.

- Thousands of women were polled by fashion magazines and asked if they loved and were happy with the appearance of their breasts. 100% of them answered that they were not. Is it any surprise that Breast Cancer is the #1 cancer in women?

- A major magazine asked a thousand people if they would rather have a different occupation. All one thousand said they would rather be doing something different. Is it any wonder Americans have the highest incidence of Cancer and Heart disease in the world?

HOW TO DO IT?

"It's GREAT to be ALIVE"

For every one little thing that you think is bad, there are 1,000 things that are *GREAT* and *WONDERFUL* about you and your life. And if you can't see the good, well, you're just not looking hard enough, or in the right place. Every day when I wake up I think about how blessed I am, how great it is to be alive and how much...

"I LOVE my LIFE"

These two great healing affirmations didn't come naturally to me.

I didn't learn them from my school teachers or hear them on television, movies or in the lyrics of songs. And I certainly didn't hear them from my patients, either. In fact, if you heard most of my patients' self-degrading, self-defeating mouths and negative minds you would wonder how they were even still

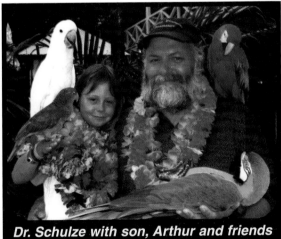

Dr. Schulze with son, Arthur and friends

alive. Imagine the kind of constant attack your immune system has to survive and defend itself against EVERY DAY. If you think flesh-eating bacteria, Legionnaire's disease and killer viral Influenzas are bad, well, medical and scientific research clearly proves that your worst immune attack, your worst immune enemy, is not microbes but what you are thinking and what comes out of your mouth, every day. Furthermore, one of the most healing nutrients to your body, more than vitamins, minerals, enzymes, fresh juices, even more than herbs, is LOVE.

HOW BAD ATTITUDES, NEGATIVE THOUGHTS, LOW SELF-ESTEEM AND A MISERABLE OUTLOOK CAUSE DISEASE

FIRST, YOUR BRAIN IS YOUR MASTER COMPUTER

Your brain is constantly working, night and day, 24 / 7 / 365; it never shuts down or takes a vacation. First off, it's your body's master computer console controlling just about every metabolic function and chemical balance in your body. From your nervous system and blood balances to your sexual function and thousands of other functions that you don't even know about, your brain is the captain at the helm, creating, driving, controlling, balancing and maintaining **YOU**, and your entire body, every second of every day.

If this doesn't sound exhausting enough, your brain also has to process everything you think. If you want to move your arm or leg, walk, run, sit, or eat or talk, your brain has to give the command and your body follows orders. To do this your brain and brain cells, just like every other cell and organ in your body, have to take in nourishment and nutrition and eliminate waste. Your brain needs this nourishment to create numerous chemicals. In fact, every time you have any thought, your brain creates a specific chemical.

Scientists now know that when you have a thought, your brain creates chemicals that open what they refer to as *windows*. And when the thought is over, the window closes. So when you see the person of your dreams and you feel love, and you have that incredible tingling feeling all over your body, this is a brain chemical. When you feel sexual, this is another brain chemical, and when that #%@&?!* cuts you off in traffic and you wish you had laser guns on your steering wheel and could vaporize this idiot, that hate, that boiling acid in your bloodstream or stomach, well that's another brain chemical. Scientists call these brain chemicals **neuropeptides**.

Science has done a lot of research on this subject for a number of reasons. Just imagine if you could put something in the water and make everyone feel loving, or more realistic, fearful, hateful, scared or numb. Medical doctors, especially psychiatrists, have also been very interested in this topic because they want to create happy and numb pills and have created many such pills already. In fact you probably know someone who is, or at least has taken, the numb pills.

What we know is when you have any thought, your brain creates chemicals which alter you, and what you feel is the creation and assimilation of these brain chemicals called *neuropeptides*.

SECOND, YOU NEED JUST A LITTLE CELLULAR ANATOMY

Your body is made up of trillions of cells: blood cells, skin cells, liver cells, brain cells. In a way you are just a bunch of cells, at least physically.

The cell wall, protective covering, membrane (or let's call it skin) forms the outer boundary of each cell. It is made up of phospholipids (fats), protein and cholesterol. ***It can selectively allow various substances to enter or leave the cell.*** In fact many substances in your bloodstream like vitamins or amino acids **have their own specific loading dock** on the cell wall where they can connect and offload their *specific* cargo. Even immune cells have these same specific loading docks on their surface skin, and now *here is where it gets weird*.

THIRD, YOU ARE WHAT YOU THINK!

Medical science made a ~~big~~, no, huge discovery in the last decade that went for the most part unnoticed. They already knew that your immune cells, just like all cells, have specific loading docks on their surfaces to assimilate particular substances. But it was discovered that on the surface of your immune cells, the cells that are designed to protect you and fight off bacteria, virus, fungus, parasites, cancer-- in fact ALL disease-- **there is a specific loading dock, a specific assimilation site, for NEUROPEPTIDES!**

What business is it to your immune cells what you are thinking? Why do they care? Don't they have enough to do with all the germs floating around these days and the cancer rate skyrocketing, without having to eavesdrop on your personal affairs and private conversations with yourself. Is this part of the new administration's war against terrorists, FBI telephone taps without warrants?

Hang on, it gets weirder. OK, so we know that your immune system is definitely listening to your emotional dialogue, but no cell, organ or system of your body listens to another system unless it is prepared to *react* to the information it is receiving. Holy bad attitude, Batman . . . does this mean . . . oh no . . . . that . . .

"Your Immune System is _LISTENING_ to and _REACTING_ to your emotional dialogue."

This is exactly what medical science is telling us now, that your immune cells have specific receptor sites for Neuropeptides, the chemicals that your brain creates with every thought, AND that your immune cells' response to germs and disease is affected, whether boosted or impaired or even STOPPED, by these brain chemicals. Your immune cells' response is determined by your thoughts.

Just think of the potential power we have to cure any disease, *or to manifest it.*

FINALLY, THE PROOF WAS IN MY CLINIC

I have always told you that in my clinic, I could tell the winners from the losers in less than 2 minutes. In other words I could tell who was going to beat their cancer, and those that weren't going to make it, almost immediately. IT WAS THEIR ATTITUDE.

I read a poll taken by a fashion magazine that asked thousands of women if they were happy with their breasts, the size, shape, and even the placement and look of their nipples. Well, every woman, ALL of them, answered NO. 100% of the women polled didn't like something about their breasts and is it any wonder that breast cancer is the #1 cancer among women? <u>Think about it</u>! Pun intended!

What I am telling you is a basic law of Newtonian physics, that "Every action has an equal reaction". There are no free rides with your mind and body connection. You are either thinking thoughts that will get you healthier and better, or you are thinking thoughts that will make you sicker and worse. In the 1960's we used to have a saying, you are either part of the solution or you are part of the problem, there is no middle ground.

What I mean is that there are physical *consequences* for everything that you do and now, it appears, for even everything that you *think* too. I am not trying to lay a guilt trip on you here. This is just the way it is.

"Your Attitude is your Altitude"

Look, I had a young woman that I was treating in my clinic that had AIDS. She had contacted me because I had a reputation of having success with helping people with AIDS actually heal themselves. I knew of her and she really had everything going for her; she was young, strong, quite healthy, but had been infected with HIV. I was actually shocked to discover that the disease had spread so rapidly in her and that she was now showing gross symptoms of AIDS, much faster than most infected with HIV, and her t-cell count had dropped to only 2, the lowest I had ever heard of, in just a few months with HIV, and she had developed a cancer!

Since many of my patients that had been infected with HIV for over a decade were very alive and very well, I was shocked with how this young woman in her prime could be so hurt by this disease so quickly, until she opened her foul mouth. I have rarely heard someone so negative in all of my life. She must have had some great training from her parents and teachers. She never had anything good to say about anything, EVER. Well, I took her on as a patient because she had so much going for her: young age, fairly healthy, etc.

In her very first office visit I mentioned her bad attitude and negative affirmations and told her that by her next visit in a week, I wanted to see and hear an attitude change and I suggested some positive affirmation reading material. Well the next week I didn't see any attitude change, she was still bummerwoman. She was taking all of her herbs, and doing all of her natural healing routines, her colon was clean but her brain was still filled with fecal matter. I told her that if she didn't come up with at least one positive affirmation by her next appointment that I would fire her as a patient. The third week she came into my clinic and said she had her first *supposed* positive affirmation. She said *"My cancer is not going to eat me alive and kill me"*. This was the best that she could do? She was dead in 2 weeks.

NEW HEALING THOUGHTS

After working in my clinic spanning 3 decades, my patients taught me a lot. But above anything else I saw that our most powerful healing tool, and our most destructive, was our mind.

In life I have also learned that if you want something, you can create it. You can manifest it. Ask and you shall receive. However you want to look at life, or health, I have learned that ANYTHING is possible.

I have patients that were told by the best of the best specialists, the heads of the hospital departments, the top at the Mayo Clinic, or Harvard or Stanford, the finest, smartest and highest educated medical doctors in the world that they would be dead in a few weeks or months, **THIRTY YEARS AGO,** and they are still very alive and very healthy today. How is this possible? Well, part of it is certainly that they were willing to change just about everything in their life. But the biggest part is that they believed that they could be well, they could see it, they could feel it, they could taste it, **AND THEN THEY CREATED IT!**

And every one of them, every one of my patients, had to learn a new positive way to look at themselves, and at life. They were forced into this by their circumstance, their disease.

For the rest of us, it is much better to make these changes before you get sick, and what better time to do this than at the beginning of a new year and a new millennium. So let's get started with our preventative emotional medicine.

YOUR BODY

At first you don't have to believe everything that you say. Just like anything, it takes a little practice. Eventually you will become a believer.

You must understand that you will never be well if you don't love yourself, so you have to start telling yourself this RIGHT NOW. You have to start creating the right brain chemicals, the right neuropeptides, to turn your immune system back on, to supercharge your immune system. Come on friends, my Echinacea Plus needs some help here.

A great affirmation, great words to start with, are "I love myself". Look into the mirror every morning and shout this out loud. Sure, you may think that you are not perfect, but who is? That is what is so great and exciting about life. We are all different, YAHOO! So look at yourself, and love yourself, and say it, say the words. Whatever you look like and wherever you are on your healing or destructive path, it all starts right here, RIGHT NOW. Be bold, take the leap, have the courage and the faith, I LOVE MYSELF. It feels good. Try it, and with a big smile, try it naked.

Sure, you may have a few parts that don't work so well. Who doesn't? That's no excuse for self hate. For every one little thing that you think is wrong with you I could find and tell you about a 1000 things that are working great that you don't even see or acknowledge.

Don't make me come over to your house and open a can of whoop ass on you, make you drop and give me twenty right now. I want you to start loving yourself today. It will take a little practice but it will make the biggest difference in your life, ever.

YOUR LIFE

Are you going to waste the greatest gift you have received from God? Are you going to blow it, are you going to sit on the sidelines and watch life pass you by chanting *"why is this happening to me?"*, or are you going to do something about it, your life, and celebrate every day and celebrate everything that comes your way? So shout it out, loud and long, and often . . . .

"It's GREAT to be ALIVE"

If there is one thing that I have learned in my clinic, and in life, it is that EVERYTHING, that's right, EVERYTHING, IS A BLESSING FROM GOD. EVERYTHING.

Sure, at the moment, and in the moment, it may be hard to see the blessing in a dead car battery, or locking yourself out of your house, a broken washing machine, a broken leg, or diabetes or a heart attack or cancer, but trust me on this one, it is your gift from God. Every patient that I ever had was eventually able to look at their disease or injury and thank God for it, the lesson, what they learned and how their disease changed their life. Diseases, injuries, whatever. . . they aren't accidents, or horrors, they are tools to learn from, lessons, in how to change our lives for the better. They are gifts. They are not bumps in the road, they are _**JEWELS**_. They are a stop sign, at a fork in the road, and now you have a choice: suffer, blame, pain and hell . . . or . . . change, responsibility, health and heaven. It is up to you.

"I LOVE my LIFE"

How dare you judge your circumstances and decide that anything is wrong, or bad, or a bummer. How dare you. How ungrateful, unfaithful and untrusting we can be. You can't see the whole picture, how this will turn out. How many stories have you heard about people who worked in the World Trade Center in New York City that broke their glasses, or spilled their coffee on their shirt, broke their leg or they were mugged or whose car broke down the morning of September 11 and they missed getting to work, or had to leave work as soon as they arrived, and their life was spared because of this so-called bad accident? I bet you every one of them was cursing and pissed off, until the planes struck the buildings.

And what about those that died? How do we really know what they experienced, or what they are experiencing right now, or what will happen to their families and what change will take place in their home, their community and in the world because of this. How do any of us know enough to doubt or judge anything that happens and decide that it is bad.

CELEBRATE EVERYTHING; that is what I have learned. When I get a flat tire, or the person in the car in front of me does, I believe that this is a very special moment, a very special gift and a wonderful opportunity, that God is speaking to me, and that I need to pay special attention, because a divine message is coming down the pipe and this is no time to be unconscious because I don't want to miss it.

And if you start thinking this way, well, eventually every day and every single moment becomes a celebration, a gift, a message, and you become more connected with life, love, God and bliss, and as my friend Bodhi says, "life becomes one big giggle," one big celebration, ALL IS WELL, ALL OF THE TIME. This is my life, it takes a little practice, and it can be yours too.

Love, Light, Laughter and Peace

P.S. OK, let's say that old Dr. Schulze is mad as a hatter. What is the downside of following what I say? <u>**Well, one thing that is for sure is that there is nothing positive or healing that will come out of being negative.**</u> Besides getting a headache or an upset stomach, you will depress your immune system. On the contrary, being positive will ease your nerves, relax your muscles, increase your blood circulation, increase your immune strength and help you sleep like a baby. This is why it is better to think of a cold as an opportunity for your body to cleanse and purify itself and your immune system to get stronger and more educated than an attack by a killer microbe.

AT THE HEART OF IT ALL
THE COMMON DENOMINATOR OF ALL RELIGION

Organized religions of the world are responsible for killing more people than every war, disease, plague, natural disaster and dictator in history, even Adolph Hitler.

On the other hand, after years of religious and philosophical study, I know that the common wish of all religions, the written word of God in any language or any religion, in all the hundreds of religious books, the message of God, the spirit of God, no matter how hard organized religions of the world try to hide it, bury it, kill it and behave badly . . . is LOVE.

Since all of these religions don't seem to agree on much, then I think that this is a very important, powerful point I am making. That . . . .

Love is the spiritual common denominator.

This leads me to the final step in my book,

LOVE

To heal yourself of any disease, any illness, to be healthy, you need to love more. Love yourself, love your kids, love your family, love strangers, love your enemies, love your life, love what you do, love your disease and love being loving and when you run out of things to love, then love running out of things to love.

I know being loving doesn't come naturally to most, that's why we have to practice it, but believe me, it is more nutritious than beets and more healing than carrot juice.

On my travels in India I heard these lyrics to a song . . . .

Love is such a beautiful feeling,
Dance till you fall in Love
Love is such a beautiful feeling,
Dance till you fall in Love
Disappear in this song,
till the dancer is gone
And till only the LOVE remains.

DR. SCHULZE DESCRIBES HIS IMMUNE SYSTEM FORMULAE

Echinacea PLUS

While you are perfecting your emotional dialogue, protect your immune system

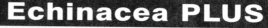

Botanical Ingredients: *Wild-harvested Echinacea angustifolia fresh root and juice, Organic Echinacea purpurea seed, Organic Garlic juice, and Organic Habanero Cayenne pepper and juice.*

Therapeutic Action: Simply put, **Echinacea** works in two main ways. First, it builds up your immune system by stimulating your body to build more immune cells and immune chemicals. Secondly, it also stimulates these immune cells into action and heightened activity levels. These actions will help you combat any infection or disease more effectively and also protect you from future invasion and illness.

Echinacea is one of the strongest immune stimulators and enhancers known. It can double and triple the amount of T-cells and Macrophages in your bloodstream and increase the number of Granulocytes. It also stimulates the phagocytosis, the ability to kill and eat the bad guys, in all of these white blood cells. Echinacea can also increase the amount of Interferon, Interleukin, Immunoglobulin and other important natural immune chemicals present in your blood. **Again, this is how Echinacea works, by boosting the number of immune cells and the amount of natural immune chemicals in your body and then stimulating them into being more active.** This is why in my clinic, Echinacea Plus was an extremely effective treatment, not only for acute infections, but also for long term diseases.

Dosage: For general maintenance use 2 droppersful (about 60 drops), three times daily. For more specific dosages see American Botanical Pharmacy catalog or call 1-800-HERB DOC.

DR. SCHULZE QUOTE: "The MAIN metabolic function of your IMMUNE SYSTEM, and your BODY, is to constantly HEAL and REPAIR itself; REPAIR you."

21 CHAPTER TWENTY-ONE

FINAL THOUGHTS

In closing, healing disease is not really that difficult. After all, even modern medicine, with its scalpels, stitches and chemical pills, achieves that. Healing just means that the diseased part is not diseased any more. Or, as with surgery, that it's completely gone. The broken part is repaired, the clogged part is unclogged. The rotten part has stopped rotting. With my twenty steps I'm offering you much more than healing. I'm offering you a new life.

See, after twenty years with sick and dying patients, I came to realize that your disease, your illness, was not bad, not the enemy, not the curse from the devil. Your disease is... WONDERFUL. That's right, I said wonderful. In fact, it's a blessing you've received from God to get your attention. To get you to change the path that you're on. Who knows, maybe just to get you to listen to me so that you can fix the disease.

Following my twenty steps you will definitely be healed. You will have a miracle. Listen to the divine message that was sent to you that brought you to my doorstep. You are being given a very special chance right here, right now. Sometimes this chance only comes once in a lifetime. A chance to not only be born and to die, but to really live. The question is, do you just want to be a healed patient, or do you want to be an ADVENTURER? A COSMONAUT? AN EXPLORER? Do you believe that there's more to living than just wading through life with a mundane spirit and a dull look on your face? God has given you an incredible gift: LIFE. Are you going to live it or are you going to sleepwalk through it? What I'm telling you is that there are many realities and I live in the one where you're laughing, loving, extremely happy, blissed out every day— no bad news, just good news. No bummers, only divine messages and divine blessings.

Follow these twenty steps and you will be healed. But learn to *live* these twenty steps. Learn to live them, and a life filled with laughter, love and light is yours. So start every day with all my steps in your heart. When you wake each morning, go over the list and each day you'll get better and better at living a healthy life. You will change and, in doing so, you will change the world.

FINAL HOUR REGRETS

In the many years I spent interviewing patients, not only in America but all over the world, I had the wonderful opportunity to talk with many elderly people. I also had the illuminating experience of being with many people just a few days, even a few hours, before their death. For a few, I was the last person they saw. I must share with you that most of these visits were filled with regrets. The reason I'm telling you this is so you don't make the same mistakes.

What I heard was like a condensed version of their life. People have a tendency near death to look back at their life and examine it. What I heard were the many regrets for not living life to its fullest.

I don't remember ever hearing any regrets for believing too much, trusting too much, laughing too much or loving too much. All the regrets were based on holding back, not going far enough, not giving enough, not loving enough, not taking the chance, not saying what they wanted to say, not taking the risk, not living life totally.

Let's not wait until it is too late. Let's not have a list of unfulfilled wishes and unlived dreams as the final hour approaches. Take the chance, take the leap, dare to make this life rich. Love and live life to its fullest potential.

What if you only had six months left to live?

What would you do differently? Who would you tell you love more? How would you spend your time? How would you live each day... each moment...

This is how I want you to live RIGHT NOW!

A POEM FROM DR. SCHULZE'S DEAD PATIENTS

We screwed up.
Don't make our same mistakes. Don't hold back.
Don't be stingy.
We all waited until it was too late
Now sitting on our death beds, gasping our last breath.

We all agree, we wasted our lives. We didn't really live.
We would do anything for a few more hours,
But all we can do is warn you,
Tell you that you are making the same mistakes we did.

We regret letting our fear and complacency rule us.
We didn't go far enough. We didn't live enough.
We didn't love enough. We didn't take enough chances.
We kept our mouths shut and didn't say what we really
wanted to say.

We should have trusted more, believed more,
Laughed more, loved more.
We should have taken more risks, lived life to the fullest,
Traveled more, worked less and had more sex.

It's too late for us. We have so many unfulfilled wishes
And so many unlived dreams.
Please don't make our same mistakes.
Take the chance. Take the leap. Love Life and Live Life
to the fullest.

DR. SCHULZE
QUOTE:

"Life is not a dress rehearsal. THIS IS IT, RIGHT NOW. You can choose to sit on the sidelines and watch it drift by, or Love and Live Life to your fullest potential."

DR. SCHULZE'S
WHERE DO I START! PROGRAM

> This program is the place to START if you don't know what to do! If you want <u>BETTER HEALTH</u> and <u>MORE ENERGY</u>, but you want it <u>CHEAP</u>, only have <u>2 MINUTES</u> and it must be <u>EASY!</u>
>
> Then this program is for you because all <u>YOU</u> have to do is swallow, and I guarantee the <u>RESULTS</u>!

MAXIMUM RESULTS
MINIMUM EFFORT

DON'T KNOW WHERE TO START?

Every patient that walked into my clinic was nutritionally depleted. A lack of nutrition in your blood can cause everything from low energy and a weak immune system to virtually any disease. Your speed and ability to recover are greatly reduced when you are nutritionally depleted. Nutrition is what builds every cell, every organ and every metabolic chemical in your body. <u>Nutrition is what builds your body; it's what YOU are made of.</u> **Having a rich supply of nutrition in your blood gives you energy, vitality, strength, protects you from disease and illness, and if you get sick, speeds up your recovery dramatically.** This is the exact program I gave to EVERY ONE of my patients that came to see me for a first visit in my clinic, EVERY SINGLE ONE OF THEM! **The program is simple. Get maximum nutrition in, get old waste out and supercharge your immune system.**

DON'T HAVE THE TIME?

For 2 decades I operated my clinic in Hollywood and Malibu, California. My patients were movie directors, producers, actors, actresses and models. They had no time, period. You can't find busier people, under more stress, living a faster paced and more hectic life. They had NO TIME and any program I put them on, at least in the beginning, had to be EASY, FAST and SIMPLE. This entire program really only takes about 2 minutes a day to prepare and do. **It doesn't get much quicker.**